e-Therapy

Case Studies, Guiding Principles, and
the Clinical Potential of the Internet

A Norton Professional Book

e-Therapy

Case Studies, Guiding Principles, and the Clinical Potential of the Internet

ROBERT C HSIUNG, Editor

W. W. Norton & Company
New York • London

For information about permission to
reproduce selections from this book, write to
Permissions, W. W. Norton & Company, Inc.,
500 Fifth Avenue, New York, NY 10110

Composition and book design by TechBooks
Manufacturing by Haddon Craftsmen
Production Manager: Leeann Graham

Library of Congress Cataloging-in-Publication Data

e-therapy : case studies, guiding principles, and the clinical potential of the Internet /
Robert C Hsiung, editor.
        p.   cm.—(A Norton professional book)
    Includes bibliographical references and index.
    ISBN 0-393-70370-3
    1. Mental health—Computer network resources.   2. Mental
illness—Diagnosis—Computer network resources.   3. Mental
illness—Treatment—Computer network resources.   4. Electronic mail systems.
    5. Internet.   6. World Wide Web.   I. Hsiung, Robert C.   II. Series.
                    RA790.5 .E2   2002
            025.06'61689—dc21   2002075331

W. W. Norton & Company, Inc., 500 Fifth Avenue, New York, N.Y. 10110
www.wwnorton.com
W. W. Norton & Company Ltd., Castle House, 75/76 Wells St., London W1T 3QT
                    1 2 3 4 5 6 7 8 9 0

Contents

Contributors   vii

Introduction: The Clinical Potential of the Internet   ix
    Robert C Hsiung

Acknowledgments   xxv

1. The Information Explosion in Mental Health   1
    Robert S. Kennedy
2. The Internet "Expert": Promise and Perils   24
    Ronald Pies
3. Using E-Mail to Support the Outpatient Treatment
of Anorexia Nervosa   39
    Joel Yager
4. A Model Community Telepsychiatry Program in Rural Arizona   69
    Sara F. Gibson, Susan Morley, Catherine P. Romeo-Wolff
5. Chat Room Therapy   92
    Gary S. Stofle
6. Clinical Principles to Guide the Practice of E-Therapy   136
    Peter M. Yellowlees
7. Suggested Principles of Professional Ethics for E-Therapy   150
    Robert C Hsiung
8. The Legal Implications of E-Therapy   166
    Nicolas P. Terry
9. My Life as an E-Patient   194
    Martha Ainsworth

Index   217

Contributors

Martha Ainsworth is Founder and Director of Metanoia.org, Community Producer for Beliefnet.com, President of the International Society of Mental Health Online.

Sara F. Gibson, M.D., is Medical Director of Telemedicine at the Northern Arizona Regional Behavioral Health Authority, and Medical Director of Little Colorado Behavioral Health Centers in Apache County, Arizona.

Robert C Hsiung, M.D., is Associate Professor of Clinical Psychiatry at the University of Chicago, and Dr. Bob at dr-bob.org.

Robert S. Kennedy, M.A., is Site Editor and Program Director of Psychiatry & Mental Health and Editor of *Technology & Medicine* at Medscape, and Associate Professor in Psychiatry at the Albert Einstein College of Medicine.

Susan Morley, M.S.W, C.I.S.W., is Director of both Telemedicine and Human Resources at the Northern Arizona Regional Behavioral Health Authority.

Ronald Pies, M.D., is Clinical Professor of Psychiatry at Tufts University, a lecturer on psychiatry at Harvard Medical School, and the expert at Mental Health InfoSource.

Catherine P. Romeo-Wolff, M.A., is the former Manager of Telemedicine at the Northern Arizona Regional Behavioral Health Authority, and currently a consultant and telecommunications agent in Flagstaff, Arizona.

Gary S. Stofle, M.S.S.W., L.I.S.W., is team leader of a Community Treatment Team in Columbus, Ohio, and Secretary of the International Society of Mental Health Online.

Nicolas P. Terry, LL.M., is Professor of Law and Codirector of the Center for Health Law Studies at Saint Louis University School of Law, Coeditor-in-Chief of *The Journal of Health Law*, and a member of the Board of Directors of the American Society of Law, Medicine & Ethics.

Joel Yager, M.D., is a professor and Vice Chair for Education in the Department of Psychiatry at the University of New Mexico School of Medicine, and Professor Emeritus in the Department of Psychiatry and Biobehavioral Sciences at the University of California, Los Angeles.

Peter Yellowlees, M.D., is Professor of Psychiatry and Director of The Center for Online Health at the University of Queensland, Australia, and Chief Scientific Officer and cofounder of Health Share Pty Ltd.

Introduction: The Clinical Potential of the Internet

Robert C Hsiung

Five curious blind men visited the palace of the Rajah to learn the truth about e-therapy. They were taken to his study, where he kept his computer (which had screen reader and voice recognition software installed).

The first blind man used a search engine to look up the side effects of Prozac. "E-therapy is comprehensive like an encyclopedia!" he declared.

The second blind man used the computer to send a question to an expert psychiatrist. "E-therapy is personal like 'Dear Abby'," he announced when he received an answer.

The third blind man e-mailed his therapist to tell her he had had another dream about elephants. "I was right," he decided. "This lets me have access to my therapist whenever I want."

The fourth blind man talked with a psychiatrist in far-off Arizona. "What we have here," he said, "is a telephone."

The fifth blind man went into a chat room and had a session with a therapist who did not know he was blind. "I believe e-therapy is like a magic carpet that takes me to a place without stigma," he said. (adapted from Blubaugh, n.d.)

It seems preposterous that e-therapy could be all these things, but different parts of it have evolved to specialize in different functions, sometimes with incongruous results. This book reflects its subject and may itself be a little ungainly, but at least it—unlike an elephant—does not weigh a ton.

Information Online

In Chapter 1, "The Information Exploration in Mental Health," Robert Kennedy provides an overview of the initial use of the Internet in mental health: to exchange information. He reviews the development of the Internet from a U.S. military project to a mass medium and addresses its both technical and sociological aspects. He discusses the two sides of information exchange: what consumers are looking for and what e-publishers like Medscape (www.medscape.com) are providing. He explains how to search effectively for information and how to assess the accuracy of the results. He concludes by looking into the future of online information, where he sees distance learning, digital health records, XML, personalization, and the lessening of information overload.

The Web is disorganized. It is an example of what could be called the Second Law of Infodynamics: Information tends toward a state of randomness (Klyce, 2001). Organization and structure require the input of energy. Kennedy refers to this as Phase II of the evolution of information transfer. Writers have to work to organize their thoughts, "Webmasters" have to work to organize their Web pages, and someone has to work to organize Web sites. Most users achieve some organization with their bookmarks. Many also rely on what Kennedy calls the "catalog" type of search engine; essentially, the bookmarks of third parties. Many people use a combination of these approaches. The more extensive—and organized—the bookmarks and the catalogs they use, and the more skilled they are at using what Kennedy calls the "index" type of search engine, the more helpful users will find the Web. Another aspect of the filtering process involves not relevance, but quality. Quality can also be assessed by users themselves or by third parties. Third parties may be biased, however, so the more information-literate users are, the better. As Terry (Chapter 8) puts it, utility is based on a series of factors: breadth of information, search efficiency, and quality of information.

Case Study: Ask the Expert

In Chapter 2, "The Internet 'Expert': Promise and Perils," Ronald Pies presents his "Ask the Expert" Web site (www.mhsource.com/expert), at which he responds publicly to questions submitted by consumers and professionals. His individualized information service is a hybrid between general information like that discussed by Kennedy (Chapter 1) and individual treatment like that provided by Stofle (Chapter 5). The key is to provide information but not advice, education but not treatment, and thereby to avoid creating a doctor–patient relationship (see Chapter 8). At most, Pies provides "heuristic," as opposed to "prescriptive" or "proscriptive," advice. The distinction is between suggesting a way to solve a problem and suggesting a solution to the problem—the classic difference between teaching someone how to fish and giving him or her a fish. There are exceptions to every rule, however, and Pies does give prescriptive and proscriptive advice in certain circumstances (e.g., when it is common sense, in cases of clear malpractice by a treating professional, and in life-threatening situations).

The site says it is "intended . . . not as a substitute for . . . urgent medical evaluation, treatment or consultation," but it falls short of saying it absolutely should not be used in crisis situations. That sort of use could be considered noncompliance, but in Chapter 6 Yellowlees tells us that the patient is becoming more autonomous, the provider–consumer relationship is becoming more egalitarian, and professionals need, in turn, to become more flexible. In his chapter, Pies demonstrates how he still does try to help in extreme situations.

Pies gives us six actual examples of questions and answers. They are mini-case studies in which he shows us not only what he does, but why he does it. He concludes by touching on the personal satisfaction he derives from this work: It is a change of pace from his usual office practice, many visitors are grateful for his help, and those efforts, as do other forms of "media psychiatry" (American Psychological Association Division 46, 2001), go much further than they would in person.

Although what Pies provides at his site is not therapy, he nevertheless uses his therapy skills. He attends not only to the questions that are submitted, but to those that are unspoken; he approaches each interaction with specific goals; he keeps in mind the real-world lives of his visitors; and he anticipates both how they might feel and what they might do in response to his replies. He is aware of both the promise and the perils of this psychoeducational form of e-therapy. He is an expert in terms of not only what he knows, but also how he deals with people.

Case Study: Adjunctive E-Mail

In Chapter 3, "Using E-Mail to Support the Outpatient Treatment of Anorexia Nervosa," Joel Yager describes how his use of e-mail has evolved from scheduling appointments to being an integral part of the treatment he provides. As more and more of his patients started to use e-mail, and especially after he moved from Southern California to New Mexico, he realized that e-mail could augment the treatment and consultation he provided. He presents cases, with e-mail transcripts, to illustrate seven ways in which e-mail may be incorporated into treatment both directly and, through consultation with other professionals, indirectly. It may be used to enhance weekly sessions, monitor treatment from a distance, monitor behavior daily, smooth a transition between care providers, communicate with family members, co-manage a patient, or intervene in a crisis. The e-mail transcripts offer concrete examples of both how patients use e-mail and how therapists can be responsive, supportive, and therapeutic using just text. This is another case of the flexibility that Yellowlees advocates.

Yager then discusses the potential positive and negative consequences of the adjunctive use of e-mail, and the possible directions future work might take. Incorporating e-mail into treatment may increase the frequency of therapist–patient contact and therefore increase the "object constancy" (Mahler, Pine, & Bergman, 1975) of the therapist. The patient may feel that the therapist is more "present" (see Chapter 5) and provides more of a "holding environment" (Winnicott, 1953). The patient may more easily initiate contact and may therefore feel both more cared about and more empowered. Because the communication is online, the patient may feel safer and therefore less inhibited (Chapters 5 and 9); because it is "asynchronous" (not in real time), the patient may worry less about possibly intruding on the therapist. The patient may engage "while the iron is hot" and thus may share more meaningful material at an earlier point in the process.

The only actual drawback Yager found was resentment at being expected to "report in." A potential drawback was getting less information via e-mail than in person but, in these cases, e-mail was an adjunct to and not a substitute for contact in person. The potential for a breach of confidentiality was the greatest with his patient A because at one point she shared a home computer, but Yager was aware of the situation and protected her privacy by taking pains to be discreet—as he would have had he met with the patient and a family member in person. Yager finds his adjunctive use of e-mail accepted by his patients and his colleagues and not too demanding of his time. He does not charge for e-mail services. Therapists could, however, bill for adjunctive online contact directly, as they do for a distinct procedure like a telephone call [Current Procedural Terminology (American Medical Association, 2001) code 99371, 99372, or 99373], or indirectly, by "bundling" it, like an office expense, into other charges.

Yager notes that patients with eating disorders tend to be compliant but shy, so they may be especially likely to make use of and to benefit from this type of e-therapy. For any patients with a behavioral problem, frequent self-reports by e-mail would help them to confront those behaviors more consistently. In general, the issue of which patients are likely to benefit from which e-therapy techniques needs more study. One size does not fit all any more online than it does in the office; even Yager was not able to engage his patients E and F by e-mail.

Case Study: Community Telepsychiatry

In Chapter 4, "A Model Community Telepsychiatry Program in Rural Arizona," Sara Gibson, Susan Morley, and Catherine Romeo-Wolff relate their experiences with NARBHA Net, the Northern Arizona Regional Behavioral Health Authority (www.rbha.net) videoconferencing system that connects—via a central hub—11 rural mental health care agencies in a 62,000-square mile area, Arizona State Hospital, the University of Arizona, the state Department of Health Services, and two other regional networks. Gibson provides all outpatient psychiatric services to one 11,000-square-mile county from the hub, which is over 150 miles away. She never meets those patients in person, yet she diagnoses their problems and prescribes their medications. She cannot assess some patients adequately that way, but she refers them to local resources, and they are no worse off than before.

One of the advantages of rural areas is that people have room to spread out. As Yager (Chapter 3) also found when he moved to Albuquerque, one of the disadvantages is that resources are more difficult to access in person. NARBHA staff sometimes used to take an entire day to attend a 30-minute meeting. Electronic communication can bridge those distances. NARBHA Net is an electronic network, but it forms the basis for human networks (see also Chapter 1) that include outpatient clinicians, inpatient clinicians, subspecialist consultants, school personnel, patient advocates, families, and, of course, patients themselves. Gibson, Morley, and Romeo-Wolff estimate that in 1998–99, 6,500 hours of staff travel time and $100,000 in expenses were saved because of NARBHA Net. And, of course, there are no automobile accidents in "cyberspace." Private insurers pay for the services provided by the telepsychiatrist at the same rate as services provided in person (but do not cover the services simultaneously provided in person by other professionals at the rural clinics). Gibson, Morley, and Romeo-Wolff found no significant differences in medication costs or hospitalization rates between the telepsychiatry patients and NARBHA patients overall.

In 1999, NARBHA Net was used for 2,200 videoconferences, 90% of which were for clinical purposes. To maximize video quality and confidentiality, they transmit at 512 kilobits per second (kbps) over private lines. A network is a many splendored thing, and NARBHA Net is also used for voice and data applications and provides educational and administrative benefits.

Feedback from both patients and staff in the rural clinics has been over-whelmingly positive. No patients have refused telepsychiatry services. In fact, the patients have tended to like telepsychiatry more than the staff has, and the price of success has been heavy demand. Gibson, Morley, and Romeo-Wolff share some tips on how to help patients "forget the machine," to make the interaction as much like interacting in person as possible, and to maximize their feeling of "presence" (see Chapter 5). They also include their consent form for others to use as a model.

Videoconferencing at 512 kbps is the next best thing to being there. Taking into account the cost of travel, it may be even better than being there. The question is, how much bandwidth is close *enough* to being there? NARBHA insisted on 512 kbps in order to administer the Abnormal Involuntary Movement Scale. If not assessing for movement disorders, however, that much bandwidth might not be necessary; one does not need the Concorde to go to the grocery store. NARBHA plans to experiment with portable telemedicine units that connect at 56 kbps (i.e., over plain old telephone service, or POTS, lines). That will be like taking the bus, but it may be good enough. POTS is already widely, if not universally, available in patients' homes, so patients will not even be tied to their local clinics. The Concorde, like the VTEL TC2000, is of more limited application not only because it is itself expensive, but also because it requires an expensive infrastructure. A bus does not need an airport. Sometimes less is more.

Case Study: Chat Room Therapy

In Chapter 5, "Chat Room Therapy," Gary Stofle reviews the use of chat rooms for individual e-therapy. He believes that to be competent at e-therapy, it is necessary, but not sufficient, to be competent at therapy in person, because "the methods of intervention must be adapted to fit the methods of communication." He discusses how both knowing who patients "really" are and protecting their confidentiality are in some ways more difficult online than in person. He also rightly points out that e-therapy should not be held to a higher standard than therapy in person. How many therapists ask the patients they see in person for identification, or have iron-clad office security?

Stofle mentions three practical ways in which chat room therapy is different from therapy in person: It is not obvious to third parties when the therapist is with the patient, so the therapist is more easily interrupted; the patient is not watching the therapist, so the therapist is more easily distracted; and the delay, even if slight, caused by having to type and to wait for transmission may lead to the therapist and the patient getting "out of synch" (as can happen on the telephone when connecting via satellite; even in person, it may take time to absorb what someone says or to formulate a response).

The heart of Chapter 5 is transcripts from three types of cases: single-session, short-term, and long-term. Stofle proves to us that psychotherapy can be done online by actually doing it. He explores, empowers, supports, gives hope, assesses suicidality, makes cognitive and behavioral interventions, elucidates psychodynamics, and interprets. We see that he can do what therapists do in person, and that it has therapeutic effects. His chat room patients share meaningful feelings, confront previously unfaced issues, and demonstrate insight.

Stofle draws a parallel between nonverbal communication in person and "nontextual" communication online. Tone of voice provides information in person, but is absent in a chat room. "Interaction tempo" provides information in a chat room, but is absent in e-mail. Word choice, however, provides information even in e-mail. It is all a matter of the degree of experiential "richness" (or technical bandwidth) of the medium. Expressive patients are easier to get to know, whatever the modality. Online, they are more "present," and therapists will have a greater sense of "presence" with them. Other patients feel safer with more distance and take longer to get to know—again, whatever the modality. Some patients may also be more expressive in one medium than another (e.g., Ainsworth in Chapter 9 writes, "I write better than I talk"). There is additionally an intersubjective factor (Stern, 1985): The better the fit is between the therapist and the patient, the more smoothly the process will proceed. Therapist selection is an issue, just as patient selection is.

A nice example of "presence" is how Stofle refers to his typing back and forth with his patients as "talking." At least to some extent, he experiences it as being with the patients in person; even reading it now in this volume, so do we.

Guiding Principles: Clinical

In Chapter 6, "Clinical Principles to Guide the Practice of E-Therapy," Peter Yellowlees says that the Internet should be integrated into real-world practice. Therapists should, for example, welcome e-mail from patients, although not unconditionally. (In Chapter 3, Yager sets a good example of this.) Yellowlees then puts forward four basic clinical principles to guide e-therapy. First, e-therapists must be *flexible* and able to integrate a wide variety of information and to work in a "24/7," global mode. Second, e-therapists must be *respectful* of patients and allow them to have a greater voice in shaping their treatments and to join with the e-therapists in more egalitarian therapeutic relationships. Third, e-therapists must be *competent* and possess both people and computer skills, be aware of their own limitations, continue to educate themselves, and contribute to the field's evidence base. Finally, e-therapists must be *responsible* and, for example, accept and even encourage requests for second opinions and the keeping of interaction transcripts. There are also potential problems online, including Internet addiction, "cyberchondria," and deception by and questionable advice from others, to which e-therapists should alert their patients.

Yellowlees uses as an example of good e-therapy practice the system at Doctor Global (www.doctorglobal.com). Automatic screening enables immediate responses to serious problems, and quality "audits" (reviews) maintain a high level of care. Yellowlees sees the accountability of e-therapists as essential and the further transition toward self-care as inevitable. Emphasis will continue to shift from professionals to self-help networks, friends, and family, and from the therapist as authority to the therapist as advisor and collaborator.

The goal of quality audits would, of course, be quality improvement, but there are two sides to every coin, and the other side of this one may be resentment by the audited therapists. We have seen this in the United States with managed care. One hopes that lessons learned from auditing costs will be applied to auditing quality.

Guiding Principles: Ethical

In Chapter 7, "Suggested Principles of Professional Ethics for E-Therapy," I discuss some of the opportunities and dangers of e-therapy. Guidelines may help both therapists and patients to chart ethical courses of treatment. I review the development of various e-therapy ethics guidelines, and present a set of suggested principles produced by a joint committee of the International Society for Mental Health Online (ISMHO) and the Psychiatric Society for Informatics (PSI). The members of the committee came from different countries and different professional backgrounds; one of the co-chairs was a patient and not a therapist. The suggested principles were intended to be broad enough to be applied internationally and to the entire continuum of e-therapy services. The development process was conducted completely online. Like NARBHA (see Gibson, Morley, & Romeo-Wolff, Chapter 4), using electronic communication to bridge the distances separating them enabled more members to participate and the work to be more continuous because members did not have to travel to collaborate in person.

There are three sets of suggested principles. The first has to do with informed consent: The patient should be informed about the process, the therapist, the potential risks and benefits, the safeguards that the therapist takes and that the patient could take, and the alternatives. The second set concerns "standard operating procedure": E-therapy should be provided within the same standard framework as therapy in person is. The therapist should be competent, legally allowed to practice (see Chapter 8), reach an agreement with the patient on the frequency and cost of services, adequately evaluate the patient, be mindful of other treatment providers, protect the confidentiality of the patient, and maintain records of the treatment. The third set deals with emergencies: The procedures to follow in an emergency should be discussed, and if the therapist and the patient are geographically separated, the therapist should identify a local backup, such as the patient's primary care physician. These principles should help guide e-therapists as they develop their practices, and e-patients as they select among them. I have established a message board to facilitate further discussion of "distance" mental health.

Guiding Principles: Legal

In Chapter 8, "The Legal Implications of E-Therapy," Nicolas Terry reviews an area that is rapidly changing and often mystifying, yet essential to understand. He defines *e-health* and *e-therapy*, respectively, as the use of technology to deliver health care services and the clinical (as opposed to the "backend," or administrative) uses in mental health. The business-to-business side of e-therapy—consulting with other clinicians—is what he considers *telepsychiatry*; its business-to-consumer counterpart is direct patient care.

Terry starts with a discussion of the impact of e-health on the overall structure of the health care system. Rather than entering the health care system at a single point, patients will now enter at multiple points. The primary care physician gatekeeper will be rendered obsolete, and regulation will also become "multipoint." For example, a state may require not only therapists in that state, but also therapists in other states who treat patients in that state, to be licensed in that state. Or, to stay within its borders, a state may require pharmacies in that state not just to require prescriptions, but prescriptions issued on the basis of "valid" doctor–patient relationships. What constitutes "valid" relationships (or the "accepted medical practices" on which such relationships might be based) is, of course, open to interpretation. Obtaining a history is cited as an example of an accepted medical practice. But what about obtaining a history over the Internet?

Terry breaks down the relevant legal issues into four groups: those having to do with regulation, the therapist–patient relationship, quality, and security and privacy. Regulatory issues include licensure, malpractice coverage, and the prescribing and dispensing of medication. Licensure is complicated because federal, state, and intrastate jurisdictions overlap; however, in interstate B2B e-therapy, licensure may be covered by specific telemedicine clauses. In interstate B2C e-therapy, telemedicine statutes do not (currently) apply. The key concept in licensure is the practice of a regulated profession. States have the power to define those professions and may include B2C e-therapy involving their residents. States also have the power to regulate those practices, for example, by requiring licenses, certificates, and so on. E-therapists may of course hope that distant states do not expend the resources to enforce their regulations, or they may press for some form of national licensure (or at least increased reciprocity among states). Although the law may (and perhaps should) lag behind technology, it does eventually adapt. Today, statutes are starting to address telemedicine; soon, they will also deal with e-medicine.

Regarding the therapist–patient relationship, one legal issue is when a therapist–patient relationship is created. Malpractice hinges on such a relationship; in its absence, a therapist is not liable for negligence. Terry states that one does not have to practice medicine to create a doctor–patient relationship, but also cites *Miller v. Sullivan* (1995), in which the court stated that "the relationship is created when professional services are rendered and accepted for the purposes of . . . treatment." Once a therapist–patient relationship has been established, a separate legal issue is informed consent, particularly regarding risks to confidentiality.

Technology will raise the quality of care even in traditional practice. We will see a decrease in medical error and, at least in theory, "administrative simplification." In e-health, quality of information is one issue. Simply linking to other Web sites may be problematic. It is more efficient than quoting or paraphrasing, but also increases the possibility of conflicts of interest and liability for the linked-to information (which, among other problems, may change without notice). Malpractice-like actions may be difficult, but fraud and dangerous products will continue to be targeted. The quality of care issue Terry focuses on is the therapist's *Tarasoff* duty (to protect third parties) when patients are potentially violent. "Forum selection" clauses may deter some litigation, but cultivating realistic patient expectations is, in his view, more likely to be effective.

Finally, Terry discusses security and privacy. Security is keeping third parties from "breaking in" and helping themselves to information; privacy is not sharing information with third parties without authorization. The Health Information Portability and Accountability Act will have a major impact in both areas, at least in the United States. Of note are the rights of patients to correct their records and to know who has accessed their records. Disclosure to public health and law enforcement officials will be more relaxed, but there will be increased responsibility for disclosures by business associates such as billing or practice management companies.

It could be argued that that the multipoint access to health care services that e-health will bring will have advantages and disadvantages analogous to the multipoint access to health information that the Web has already brought (see Chapter 1). Among the references in Chapter 8 are links to the e-health and legal literature, and many also include links to the Web. Although it is in only "plain" text in this volume, Chapter 8 is hypertext in spirit. (Readers unfamiliar with legal citations may take advantage of the parallel information explosion in the law and consult online guides such as that provided by the Boston College Law Library, 1999.)

A Patient's Perspective

In Chapter 9, "My Life as an E-Patient," Martha Ainsworth starts with a review of the history of e-therapy, which she considers, more narrowly than Terry, to include only ongoing dyadic relationships in which all interactions are online. She believes both the advent of the dot-com e-clinics and the formation of ISMHO to be milestones in the evolution of e-therapy. Both were in fact developmental or evolutionary steps in that they involved individuals coming together to form organizations.

She then tells us about her own e-therapy. In some ways, her story is like that of a traditional therapy patient. She was in pain, and she was alone. She shopped around for a therapist. She wondered whom she could trust. She chose someone and, luckily, they clicked. She was not instantly cured, but she was no longer alone and now had hope.

Her e-therapist established a therapeutic frame (Bleger, 1967). Ainsworth held back (i.e., resisted). He sensed her moods (i.e., was empathic). Their relationship deepened. He made comments; he interpreted. There was transference, and there was healing. In other ways, it was very different from therapy in person. Connecting from the safety of her home (or at least her hotel room) and free from her therapist's physical presence, Ainsworth felt more secure, was less inhibited, and got more quickly to the heart of the matter. The process was more user-friendly; she "talked" to him when she wanted, she "listened" to him when she wanted, and she didn't have to do both at the same time. Granted, more user-friendly is not necessarily more therapeutic, but it is at least an example of the flexibility that Yellowlees advocates.

Ainsworth went on to establish Metanoia.org, to share what she had learned with others (i.e., to use the Internet to provide information). First, she created a directory of e-therapists. She also conducted a survey and presents some of that data here. Her sample was self-selected. Of 619 responses collected over 4 years, 73% had already tried e-therapy. Of those, 68% had never been in any kind of therapy before, 92% thought their e-therapy had helped, and 64% went on to try therapy in person. That 68% tried e-therapy before therapy in person shows that it appealed to some individuals. That 92% considered it helpful, but 64% went on to therapy in person, is interesting. Without more complete data, it is hard to know whether the e-therapy glass was more empty (64% did not stay with e-therapy) or more full (64% were willing, after the more user-friendly e-therapy experience, to try therapy in person).

Ainsworth became alarmed by some of the responses she received and some of the e-therapy practices she found, and decided not just to direct patients toward e-therapy but also to guide both them and e-therapists down the trail she and her own e-therapist had blazed. In Chapter 9, she discusses the appropriateness of e-therapy, the competence (see Chapters 5 and 6) and accessibility of the e-therapist, the cost of the e-therapy, and the privacy of the e-patient.

Finally, Ainsworth reflects on the evolution of e-therapy and notes that the question has shifted from *whether* e-therapy should be provided to *how*. Which e-therapists, for example, should treat which e-patients? She does not claim that "true" psychotherapy can take place online, and merely states that whatever it is called, it can be tremendously helpful and will continue to be demanded. Ainsworth's pragmatic wish is that therapists who are qualified will provide e-therapy. She appeals to other patients to speak out, and to mental health professionals to listen. The voices of patients may be softer online, coming from behind the "anonymity shield" and across the gulf of cyberspace, so therapists not only need to listen, but to listen closely.

Discussion

"E-therapy is like an encyclopedia," said the first blind man. "Surely we can agree on that."

"An encyclopedia? E-therapy is 'Dear Abby!'" answered the second blind man.

"It's an extra session, I tell you," insisted the third blind man.

"I'm certain it's a telephone," said the fourth blind man.

"Magic carpet. There's no doubt," said the fifth blind man.

Their argument continued and their shouts grew louder and louder. "Encyclopedia!" " 'Dear Abby!' " "Having a session whenever I want!" "Telephone!" "Carpet!"

"STOP SHOUTING!" called a very angry voice.

Licensure (and regulation in general) can be a contentious issue. Stofle urges us "not to recreate barriers to treatment that the Internet has eliminated." Terry explains how licensure affects e-therapy, but takes it as a given and does not attempt to justify it. The current crazy quilt of state requirements is, of course, inconvenient for e-therapists who would like to be able to treat patients from coast to coast. Licensure, like a guard rail, does, however, serve a purpose. Overregulation would of course be undesirable, like just closing the highway. But if the guard rail is removed while the highway is being upgraded to a superhighway, it *should* be replaced—as soon as it can be decided where exactly to locate it, because traffic patterns might change. It may be paternalistic, but sometimes "pater" does know best.

Gibson, Morley, and Romeo-Wolff found that patients like telepsychiatry more than the staff does. Terry observed that more e-therapy Web sites were run by masters-level therapists and clinical psychologists than by psychiatrists. We might speculate that in terms of the number of "early adopters" (Rogers, 1995) of e-therapy, there might be more patients than masters-level therapists, more masters-level therapists than clinical psychologists, and more clinical psychologists than psychiatrists. Perhaps psychiatrists as a group are the most conservative, or perhaps they benefit the most from the current system and thus have the least incentive to change.

A number of authors contributing to this volume comment on the tradeoffs of e-therapy. Ainsworth (Chapter 9) felt more comfortable communicating by e-mail: "I could reveal to him only as much as I felt comfortable revealing," and "The anonymity shield of cyberspace made me feel free." Anonymity is powerful partly because of the shame and stigma that is still—although thankfully not to the same extent as before—associated with mental illness and mental health treatment. Ainsworth's therapist may not, however, have felt so comfortable; in his very first e-mail, he started asking to talk to her on the telephone. Even after they had established a solid connection and had not only talked on the telephone but met in person, she still felt more comfortable online. Not only is less information about the patient available to the therapist under such circumstances, but less information about the therapist is available to the patient, and, as Terry points out, the therapist may seem less warm or, in Stofle's terms, less "present." Because meeting in person almost always means that the patient goes to the therapist, meeting online, in more neutral territory, is an example of the more egalitarian therapist–patient relationship to which Yellowlees refers. Terry warns that if patients have more autonomy, they may behave in more manipulative ways. Being flexible (as recommended by Yellowlees), however, the therapist might simply use that manipulation as grist for the therapeutic mill—as he or she might if treating the patient in person.

Ainsworth was not truly anonymous; her therapist knew who she was. The online "anonymity shield" does, however, raise concerns. One of the suggested ethical principles I discuss is that therapists should not be anonymous. But what about patients? I refer to it as an unresolved issue. If people are allowed to remain truly anonymous, they may feel even safer and more willing to open up. This phenomenon is apparent in online communities like Psycho-Babble (www.dr-bob.org/babble). What difference does it make if the therapist does not know the patient's name? It is not an issue of contacting the patient, because the therapist would have the patient's e-mail address (it might change, but so might the patient's telephone number). One issue is that the patient, by remaining anonymous, shifts the balance of power in the therapist–patient relationship; now the patient knows who the therapist is, but the therapist does not know who the patient is. This may be appealing to the patient, given the underlying power differential in other respects.

This shift in power also has significant consequences in *Tarasoff* situations. If the therapist does not know who the patient is, the patient is also "safe" from involuntary hospitalization. Stofle's stance is that e-therapists need to accept that they are powerless in the face of determinedly suicidal patients. Presumably, the courts should also see e-therapists as powerless (i.e., impose no *Tarasoff* duty on them). Therapists were only held liable for the death of Tatiana Tarasoff because she was "readily identifiable" as the potential victim (*Tarasoff v. Regents*, 1976). If a patient tells a therapist that he or she intends to go to a random park and shoot a random person, the therapist may be responsible for hospitalizing the patient or notifying the police, but not for warning the victim. Stofle is clear that the e-therapist should recommend appropriate treatment and decline to participate in inappropriate treatment. Perhaps the e-therapist should not be held responsible for protecting the patient from *self*-harm if the *patient* is not readily identifiable. The parallel would be with an anonymous patient who calls a hotline or an emergency room. It may be possible to identify the e-patient with the cooperation of his or her Internet service provider, but if efforts like that may be made, the patient should be informed in advance.

A more restrictive approach would be along the lines of the ISMHO/PSI suggested principles: The e-therapist might know the patient only by a pseudonym, but a local backup who knows the patient's name should be involved and could try to hospitalize the patient involuntarily, if necessary.

Alternatively, it could simply be considered unacceptable for e-therapists to treat anonymous patients. That, however, would not demonstrate the flexibility that Yellowlees encourages.

Practically speaking, to a large extent the patient identity problem will be solved online as it is in person: as a byproduct of having to pay for services. To pay, the patient will need, at least in the near term, a credit card; unless it is stolen, the credit card will identify the patient. Stofle takes checks and uses PayPal (www.paypal.com), so a checking account can be the source of funds, but a checking account also identifies the patient, and PayPal divulges the name of the payor to the payee. Online, one member of a household could pose as another, because access to a credit card or a checking account might be shared, and such a deception might be impossible in person, but at least the household would be identified.

Security may be worse online in some ways, but it may be better in others. Communicating using a Web-based secure sockets layer (SSL) system is both secure and, because most Web browsers have SSL built in and no extra software needs to be installed, user-friendly. Encrypting transmissions from one person to another is a challenge, because the "key" must also be transmitted (and therefore itself is vulnerable to interception). When one encrypts information for one's own use, however, neither the information nor the key needs to be transmitted, so the process is much more straightforward. As well, encrypted patient files may be *more* secure than paper files locked in a desk.

As Yellowlees advises, e-therapy must pick up where traditional therapy leaves off. It may, however, offer even more potential than he envisions. The issue of anonymous patients has been addressed earlier. What about answering questions "in a booth at a fair"? That smacks more of reading tea leaves than of modern evidence-based best practices. Yet, as Kennedy discusses, access to information online has clearly been a boon to patients. Patient may now Ask Jeeves (www.askjeeves.com), and Pies is an expert in a sort of virtual booth. Pies does not, however, respond in "real time." If someone like him did, would that not also be a valuable service? AmericasDoctor (www.americasdoctor.com) used to make practitioners available in chat rooms.

What about an AmericasExpert? What matters is not the setting (hospital, fair, or Internet), but the quality of the service.

> It was the Rajah, awakened from his nap by the noisy argument. "How can each of you be so certain you are right?" asked the ruler.
>
> The five blind men considered the question. And then, knowing the Rajah to be a very wise man, they said nothing at all.
>
> "E-therapy is very large," said the Rajah kindly, as he sat down at the computer. "Each man touched only one part. Perhaps if you put the parts together, you will see the truth. Now, let me surf in peace."

References

American Medical Association. (2001). CPT (current procedural terminology) [Online]. Available: www.ama-assn.org/ama/pub/category/3113.html

American Psychological Association Division 46. (2001). Media psychology [Online]. Available: www.apa.org/divisions/div46

Bleger, J. (1967). Psycho-analysis of the psycho-analytic frame. International Journal of Psycho-Analysis, 48(4), 511–519.

Blubaugh, D. (n.d.). The blind men and the elephant [Online]. Available: www.peacecorps.gov/wws/guides/looking/story22.html

Boston College Law Library. (1999). Reading legal citations [Online]. Available: www.bc.edu/bc_org/avp/law/lawlib/GUIDES-H/legalcite.html

Klyce, B. (2001). The second law of thermodynamics [Online]. Available: www.panspermia.org/seconlaw.htm

Mahler, M., Pine, F., & Bergman, A. (1975). The psychological birth of the human infant. New York: Basic.

Miller v. Sullivan. 214 A.D.2d 822, 823 (N.Y. App. Div. 1995) [Online]. Available: media.law.unimelb.edu.au/ehealth/Cases/Miller_Sullivan.htm

Rogers, E. M. (1995). Diffusion of innovations (4th ed.). New York: Free Press.

Stern, D. N. (1985). The interpersonal world of the infant: A view from psychoanalysis and developmental psychology. New York: Basic Books.

Tarasoff v. Regents of the University of California, 17 Cal.3d 425, 551 P.2d 334 (Cal. 1976).

Winnicott, D. W. (1953). Transitional objects and transitional phenomena; a study of the first not-me possession. International Journal of Psycho-Analysis, 34, 89–97.

Acknowledgments

I would like to express my deep appreciation to A. Deborah Malmud, my editor at W. W. Norton, who saw this book through from conception to delivery; Jason C. Bartz, who generated the curves for the jacket illustration; David Sommers, who provided valuable assistance; Morton M. Silverman and Elliot S. Gershon, who have steadfastly supported both my online and "real world" work; and my wife, Ingrid, who always has been loving—and cleaned up after me (even when it came to this project).

e-Therapy

Case Studies, Guiding Principles, and
the Clinical Potential of the Internet

1

The Information Explosion in Mental Health

Robert S. Kennedy

IN OUR BIOLOGICAL DEVELOPMENT, the first thing that we crave after the essentials of food and shelter is information. We are a curious species, and we have gone and will go to great lengths to seek new information. As a civilization, we have spent years constructing ways to generate or discover new information. We seem to have an unquenchable curiosity for new information and novel ways to use previous knowledge.

When the Internet was conceptualized, it was devised as a way to communicate information, originally military information and later scientific information. Unlike the telephone, it was not limited in the types of information it could transfer, and it also allowed many-to-one relationships because it was a network.

With the advent of the World Wide Web, the quantity and quality of information increased dramatically. We are a very visual culture. The ease of adoption of the Internet after the Web came about was quite dramatic—probably because of its multimedia capabilities.

The Internet and the World Wide Web

Introducing or trying to offer an explanation of the Internet is a little like trying to describe what psychotherapy is. It really is something that needs to be experienced rather than described. (Warren, Kramer, Hyler, & Kennedy, 1997)

1

FIGURE 1.1
MAJOR COMPONENTS OF THE INTERNET.

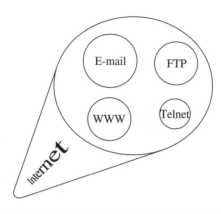

In brief, the Internet was devised in 1969 as a "network of networks" by the Advanced Research Projects Agency (ARPA) of the U.S. Department of Defense. The original ARPAnet was created to allow easy and secure communication among computers in various cities with the provision that even if some of the cities could not communicate, the others would still be able to.

The brilliance of this new network was the standardization of addresses and protocols for communicating packets of information. The communicating computers—not the network itself—were given the responsibility for ensuring that the communications were accomplished. These standards still exist today.

The World Wide Web is the fastest-growing segment of the Internet but, contrary to popular belief, it is only one segment. Other salient functions of the Internet include: the exchange of e-mail, which is still its most common use; file transfer using file transfer protocol (FTP), which is the fastest method; and telnet, which is the interface originally developed for the Unix operating system in which the user's computer functions as a simple terminal from which to run programs on other computers. Telnet is still being used to access certain databases and by systems that have not yet upgraded to a Web interface (see Figure 1.1).

The Web as a Medium

Language serves not only to express thoughts, but to make possible thoughts which could not exist without it. (Russell, 1948)

The ARPAnet was not user-friendly. Only when Tim Berners-Lee devised an attractive, easy-to-use interface for the Internet did it become a popular medium. Part of the magic of the Web is the hypertext (meaning "beyond text") links that allow linking and movement to related text or graphics regardless of their physical location. The only holdover from the Unix world that is still part of the visual Web is the structure of the addresses or uniform resource locators (URLs). The long URLs with slashes are part of the language of Unix, in which slashes separate levels of subdirectories on computers.

The only part of the Internet some people know is the Web, and its adoption into popular culture is probably due to the fact that television has made us visually oriented. Whereas TV is a passive medium, the Web has introduced a new element to information transfer: interactivity. For the first time in the history of "mass media," there is two-way communication. People can now choose what information they want and where to go for it.

The goal is information. Although television and radio have become entertainment media primarily and information sources secondarily, the Web is an "information server" primarily. The traditional media have therefore positioned the Web as an information extension. Although their typical news reports give sound bites, they offer more and, in addition, provide an interactive experience on their Web sites. This provides an opportunity for viewers to access more of the story and to navigate the information to whatever depth they desire. In previous decades, it took numerous hours of research to "discover" the additional facts of a story.

It is not just the traditional media, of course, that publish information online. The global technological psyche has changed to match the "will of the people." Although publishing a book on paper remains seductive, the average person can now publish anything he or she wishes on the World Wide Web.

Recently, the novelist Stephen King made a novella available online. It received 250,000 download requests in the first few hours. By comparison, a publisher's "best seller" only needs to sell 6,000 copies to be considered successful. This medium has truly changed the traditional world of publishing and created a new landscape. New rules are being written as the ink on old ones dries. The enterprise has morphed.

From the early days of the Internet, science has grasped onto it as an information tool, and the Web has provided an easy-to-navigate way to disseminate knowledge.

Men of science should then turn to the massive task of making more accessible our bewildering store of knowledge. For many years inventions have extended man's physical powers rather than the powers of his mind. . . . Now . . . instruments are at hand which, if properly developed, will give man access to and command over the inherited knowledge of the ages. ("Editor's Introduction," 1945)

Types of Information Online

Because the Web is such a flexible medium, the types of information that are available are as rich and varied as the human imagination can devise. The only caveat is "reader beware." Data can come from varied sources, some reliable, some not.

Online information in health and mental health can be generally divided into information for consumers and information for professionals.

Information for Consumers

A massive amount of information geared toward the consumer has been made available online over the last decade. In particular, special interest groups offer Web sites, newsgroups, mailing lists ("listserves"), and other discussion forums centered around particular mental illnesses to present information, education, and support to patients and families of patients. Through resources such as these, people with bipolar illness, schizophrenia, or Tourette's—and patients' families—can gain access to a world of sophisticated information and support.

WHAT KINDS OF INFORMATION DO CONSUMERS SEEK ONLINE?
One of the first studies evaluating the Internet and its influence on online health information seekers, the Pew Internet & American Life Project (2000), reported that 52 million American adults, or 55% of those with Internet access, had used the Web to get health or medical information. A majority of them had gone online at least once a month for health information. A great many health information seekers said the resources they found on the Web had a direct effect on the decisions they made about their health care and on their interactions with doctors.

Specifically, of the 21 million health information seekers who said they were swayed by what they read online the last time they had sought health information:

- 70% said the Web information had influenced their decision about how to treat an illness or condition.

- 50% said it had led them to ask a doctor new questions or to get a second opinion from another doctor.
- 28% said it had affected their decision about whether or not to visit a doctor.

MORE INFORMATION ABOUT ILLNESS THAN WELLNESS

The Internet is a tool for those who are already sick more than for those who want to stay well:

- 91% of health information seekers had looked for material related to a physical illness.
- 26% had looked for mental health information.
- 13% had sought information about fitness and nutrition.
- 11% had sought basic news about health care.
- 9% had sought information about specific doctors, hospitals, or medicines.

According to the survey, the Internet was also used by family members to seek help for ailing loved ones. A great many were using the Web to gather information. Fifty-four percent of health information seekers said they were searching for information on behalf of someone else, including their children, their parents, and other relatives, during the most recent time they went online for health information.

Regarding the question of why health information seekers liked the Internet, their responses made it clear that they appreciated the convenience of access at any hour, the wealth of information available, and the ability to do research anonymously:

- 93% of health information seekers said it was important that they could get health information when it was convenient for them.
- 83% said they could get more health information online than from other sources.
- 80% said it was important to them that they could get this information without having anyone know.
- 16% said they had used the Web to get information about a sensitive health topic about which it was difficult to talk.

Finally, when surveyed about issues of privacy, respondents in the Pew project revealed that they were very anxious to have their privacy protected. They were afraid that Web sites would sell or give away information about them and that their employers or insurance companies would learn what they had done online and make decisions based on that information.

INFORMATION IS CREATING MORE SOPHISTICATED CONSUMERS

Empowering the consumer has changed the clinical relationship. Knowledge-able patients are visiting clinics and doctors' offices armed with more informa-tion and asking more sophisticated questions. Unfortunately, this also has a negative side, as some have gathered from noncredible sources data that need to be corrected by the clinician.

Information for Professionals

Professionals are seeking different information online than are consumers, al-though they are also interested in what their patients are reading and learning. Professionals seek and demand greater depth and scientific accuracy from ma-terial online. After the ARPAnet was converted into the Internet, the foremost activity on the Internet was the exchange of academic and research information among universities.

NATIONAL LIBRARY OF MEDICINE AND UNIVERSITY SITES

One type of online resource is access to the scientific literature. The National Library of Medicine and universities now make their library catalogs available online, and that has changed how professionals search for information. The National Library of Medicine's (NLM) Medline is clearly the most complete and easiest-to-use database of published material in many areas of medicine and health. It is also free to access, although paper reprints must be purchased. The Cochrane Library of evidenced-based medicine is also available online.

Resources often available through university libraries include Ovid and PsycInfo. There is often a cost associated with their use. The thirst for having everything available online—and having it in its entirety (the "full text")—is now a driving force in the further development of data access and will be for decades to come. Universities are also making some of their academic pro-grams available online. These programs range from medical school curricula to residency training and fellowship offerings. Some are developing online grand rounds programs as text or as "webcasts" (video). Online programs have expanded the reach of the universities that gave birth to continuing education.

PROFESSIONAL ASSOCIATION AND PUBLISHER SITES

Professional associations and publishers compile Web sites geared toward spe-cialty groups, with ways to earn continuing education credit, clinical resources and guidelines, news, conference and meeting information, opportunities for professional development, and access to subscription journals and databases. Professional associations also offer education geared to consumers, including information about mental health issues and on how to choose a psychiatrist or psychologist.

MEDICAL MEGASITES

There are a number of new-generation medical megasites (such as Medscape, with which I am associated) that offer a vast array of medical and mental health information for professionals. Sites such as these are leading the information revolution in health and mental health, and have set the standard for making information of many types available. For example, they may offer specialty news and important announcements or advisories; for example, regarding the recall or change in labeling of a particular drug, treatment updates, original articles, conference reports, journal scans, online textbooks, peer-reviewed e-journals, "Ask the Expert" areas, clinical case conferences, discussion forums, content purchased from other professional publishers, and links to consumer sites (see Table 1.1).

Such megasites, like many professional association sites, offer special sections for members that often include access to special information and continuing education. Most of the megasites do not charge for access, but many require registration that allows the sites to track the types of information that the professionals seek most often.

If popularity is the measure, the future of the megasites is assured. Sites such as these offer quality and depth of information while presenting a wide range of clinical material and resources.

Making Information Available

Evolution of Information Transfer

From the beginning of time, the communication of important information has been the domain of specialists: shamans, healers, and physicians. At first, information transfer was direct. Knowledge was communicated visually and verbally in one-to-one relationships. Apprenticeship allowed specialized information to be passed down accurately. Next, this special knowledge was passed along using the written word. Information transfer became indirect. The early writings on parchment were the first communications that were one to many and also could be preserved over time. The value of information became clear, and libraries were built to give information a special place. The cherished apprenticeship process continued as the best way to learn complex skills. Meetings, rounds, grand rounds, and conferences allowed for a greater

TABLE 1.1
Comparison of Published Media

TRADITIONAL PRINT MEDIA	TRADITIONAL CD-ROM	PROFESSIONAL ASSOCIATION/ PUBLISHER SITES	MEDICAL MEGASITES
Fee	Fee/subscription	Subscription	Free with registration
Full text	Full text	Full text	Full text
Linear	Linear/nonlinear	Linear/nonlinear	Linear/nonlinear
Reprint (academic copies)	Printable	Printable	Printable
	Searchable	Searchable	Searchable
	Able to be cut and pasted	Able to be cut and pasted	Able to be cut and pasted
	Interactive	Interactive	Interactive
	Hypertext references	Hypertext references + Link to Medline + Link to topics in journal	Hypertext references + Link to Medline + Link to topics + Link to related articles + Link to related news + Link to other reports + Link to consumer sites + Link to entire Web
		Treatment updates Discussion forums	Treatment updates Discussion forums Original articles Conference reports Journal scans Online textbooks E-journals "Ask the Expert" areas Case conferences E-mail notification Faxback services Audio formats
Static images/ graphics	Graphics (sizeable)	Graphics (sizeable)	Graphics (sizeable)
			Video Webcasting

TABLE 1.1
(*continued*)

TRADITIONAL PRINT MEDIA	TRADITIONAL CD-ROM	PROFESSIONAL ASSOCIATION/ PUBLISHER SITES	MEDICAL MEGASITES
		E-mail table of contents	E-mail table of contents, news, new features
			Download of programs for Palm devices
		Link to publisher-specific purchases	Link to bookstore
			Physician Web sites Evolving media + Video on demand + Teaching materials + Clinical decision support + Learning the user (personalized pages) + Interactive practice guidelines & algorithms

number of people to share ideas and new knowledge. The current evolutionary step is from printed text to electronic text.

PHASE I: ACCUMULATION
In the initial scramble to offer information online, publishers simply converted traditional articles, journals, books, and so on to online formats. Text was just copied into templates with hypertext markup language (HTML) codes to format it for Web browsers. Although this enabled online access to important information, it fell short of using the full power of the Web.

PHASE II: STRUCTURE
Although accumulation was not difficult, publishers and readers alike soon realized that there needed to be much more planning and organization. The next enhancement of online material took into account the way people interacted with Web pages. Value was added by organizing the material into sections that were easier to manage and incorporating hypertext links to Medline or other material on the same topic.

PHASE III: EXTENSION

In this phase, the boundaries of the Internet will be extended beyond text and also to the desktop. As bandwidth increases, animation, video, and other types of multimedia will become more integrated. As more clinical information becomes available online, interactive programs using practice guidelines, treatment algorithms, and clinical vignettes will change the style and scope of education. Students will access online hyperlinked multimedia textbooks, and learn and enhance their skills more effectively and at their own pace.

The Internet will also extend to the computer's desktop. Information will be gathered from the Internet and delivered to the desktop without an intermediary Web browser. One current example is enhanced music-CD-player software. After you insert a music CD, it lists only "Track 1," "Track 2," and so on. If you are connected to the Internet, however, you have the option of accessing the online CDDB music database and retrieving the names of the tracks, learning more about the artists, and reviewing other works by them. As we know, the entertainment industry often drives innovation. A clinical example would be having access at the point of care to patient data in the form of digital health records (see later discussion). A physician, while with a patient, could obtain crucial diagnostic or treatment data with a mouse click. Instructions could also be retrieved, printed out, and given to the patient. None of this valuable and sometimes time-sensitive data needs to reside on the physician's computer.

PHASE IV: UNIVERSALITY

With the proliferation of mobile computing, smaller chunks of data are being requested. The final phase of the transition to electronic information transfer will involve universal access. The physician will access the patient's records and extract concise, accurate information via cell phone. If we need data, we will get it from our desktop, our personal digital assistant, or even our refrigerator. As we enhanced plain text with HTML for Web pages, we will embed it in WML (wireless markup language) for wireless devices. The issue will not be getting the information, but, as Marshall McLuhan predicted, the information itself. The device or "machine" won't matter; the information will.

E-Publication

There is a sign in a print shop that says, "We can do it fast, we can do it cheap, we can do it well. Choose any two." Readers are demanding all three of the Web.

Accuracy + speed = credibility. In the print world, except for the news media, the emphasis is on *accuracy*. Time is taken to put health-related material together and to process it through the checkpoints of editorial refinement, peer review, and attention to relevance. For a journal, the time frame from submission to publication is generally a year, occasionally less but often more.

The Internet has changed the face of publishing. Many traditional journals have electronic versions for subscribers, and a new breed of exclusively electronic e-journals is blossoming on the Web. Online, the emphasis is on *speed*. Online publishers do not have to place ink on paper—or to deliver it—and their review processes are often set up to be quick. They offer shorter publishing cycles and faster turnaround. Less attention may therefore be paid to accuracy. If a site is that of a reputable professional association or an established publisher, a reader can generally assume that its information is accurate. However, anyone can publish on the Web, and numerous other sites have sprung up that offer professional or consumer information. Professionals are generally more able than consumers to assess the accuracy of clinical information. They should know what is being presented to consumers and evaluate sites before recommending them.

STANDARDS
A number of groups are working to establish guidelines for Internet publications. According to Baur and Deering (2000), "The pervasiveness of the Internet and the World Wide Web in health and health care raises multiple concerns about privacy, confidentiality, quality assurance, professionalism, liability, and responsible medical practice." They discussed the current approach of encouraging "voluntary codes of conduct and industry self-regulation, in conjunction with selective government intervention in specific categories of unlawful activities, such as deceptive trade practices and illegal sales of prescription medications." Government regulation has been proposed and industry has responded to public concerns by creating multiple codes, guidelines, and principles for Web-based health activities.

BUILDING A READERSHIP
How do people let others know about their great Web sites? Because there is no single master directory, the most important way to help people find a site is to list it with search engines. Most catalog-type search engines offer people the opportunity to submit a Web site for inclusion. Completing a form that specifies the URL, scope, and purpose of the site does not, however, guarantee that it will be listed. Catalogs have staff who review and evaluate the site and either accept or reject it. Most sites are included unless they are amateurish and poorly constructed. Catalogs appear not to make value judgments based

on the content of the sites. There are also services that, for a fee, submit Web sites to a number of catalogs at the same time.

Another method of getting the word out is to advertise in print publications. Advertising a site in a frequently read professional newsletter, journal, or supplement lets people know that the site exists.

Journal or other publisher sites can use electronic tables of contents to take a more active approach and give readers the option of receiving, by e-mail, the contents of each new issue when it comes out. Other sites have extended this practice to notifications of new online (rather than in print) information.

Finally, word of mouth still works. People are enthusiastic about new Web sites and tell their friends and colleagues about them. This ancient and fundamental mode of information transfer should not be underestimated, even in this electronic age.

Finding Information

The Problem With Information

According to Wurman (1999), "A weekday edition of *The New York Times* contains more information than the average person was likely to come across in a lifetime in seventeenth-century England" (p. 32). Today, the success and survival of many companies depends on their ability to "locate, analyze, and use information skillfully and appropriately" (Horton, 1983, p. 15). The volume of information that we generate has certainly exceeded our ability to find, review, and understand it. Murray (1996) estimated that "in every 24-hour period approximately 20,000,000 words of technical information are being recorded. A reader capable of reading 1,000 words per minute would require 1.5 months, reading 8 hours every day, to get through 1 day's technical output, and at the end of that period, he would have fallen 5.5 years behind in his reading!" More information is now produced than at any other time in history. Over 9,000 periodicals are published in the United States each year, and almost 1,000 books are published daily around the world (Hubbard, 1987). The term *information explosion* seems quite appropriate.

Information Literacy

People and businesses are demanding more details, and our technology is providing them. Fine (1982) noted that "technology is volume—a greater number of data, more materials, more items, more detail. The result is that sometimes we are provided with both useful and useless information, and we must learn quickly to sort and choose" (p. 209).

Horton (1983) described information literacy as "involving understanding as to how computers can help identify, access, and obtain data and documents needed for problem solving and decision making" (p. 16). We need to develop information literacy to gain more control over data in all of its variations.

The Magic of Search Engines

Imagine walking into a library and being able to access not only the card catalog to locate a book, but also to access the book and even the specific chapter, page, and paragraph in which you were interested. The World Wide Web is both the best collection of the world's information that we have ever known and the worst information repository in the world. It is estimated that there are billions of Web pages and only 20% of them are indexed. The sheer volume of material and the lack of an overall index make it difficult to find the specific information you want.

> *Knowledge is of two kinds. We know a subject ourselves, or we know where we can find information upon it. (Samuel Johnson, as quoted in Boswell, 1791/1987, p. 312)*

To find information on the Web, either you have to know the exact URL at which it resides or you must search for it. How easy is it to conduct such a search? The U.S. Digital Library Initiative gave a very simple answer to this question: "The Internet is like a library without a card catalog" (Pool, 1994, p. 21). A variation of this could read: "The Internet is like a library where somebody has taken all the books off the shelves, torn their covers off, and thrown them randomly on the floor."

Why is this? Because there is a central registry of Web sites and domain names but not one of the contents of the sites, organizing the Web is quite a challenge. Also, because the Web is so open, anyone can publish anything he or she wishes, so information comes from many sources. Trying to locate information on a topic can lead to someone's doctoral dissertation or someone else's poem, and they can be considered equally relevant by search engines. Not only is one probably more relevant in a particular case, but which one is more relevant can vary. Two people searching for information on the same topic will quite possibly seek different aspects of the data. One might want the dissertation, the other the poem.

It is interesting to note that when you "search the Web," you are not searching it directly. It is impractical to search the WWW directly. The Web is the totality of all Web pages, on computers all over the world. Your computer does not search them all directly. What it actually does is search one of several intermediate databases that contain information about Web pages. Search engines are statistical systems. Their search algorithms estimate each page's probable relevance and provide you with hypertext links to them. It is only when you click on these links that your computer goes to the servers around the world to retrieve the particular documents, images, sounds, and so on that you select.

Categories of Search Engines

The Web provides four primary ways to search for content: indices, catalogs, hybrids, and metasearch engines. Indices are produced by "Web crawlers," "spiders," or "bots" (short for "robots"), all of which are automated programs that roam the Web from site to site. On each page they come to, they index every word and follow every link. Unfortunately, searching the huge databases that are produced can result in millions of pages, relevant as well as irrelevant. Using indices requires an understanding of search techniques (see later discussion) in order to conduct refined searches.

Catalogs are created by people rather than programs. A site administrator wishing his or her site to be listed submits its URL and other information about it. The catalog lists only the site as a whole, not every individual page. Catalogs typically do not later check to see if the content of the site changes.

The structure of every catalog differs, making searching inconsistent from one to another. For example, in one catalog, the category "health" may contain sites on medicine, homeopathy, health care, and fitness. In another, the category "medicine" may include sites on health and alternative medicine but not health care, and fitness sites may be classified under "lifestyle." Dedicated search sites and portals often predefine many categories to help you organize and refine searches.

Hybrids are indices that catalog their information as well. Metasearch engines do not use their own databases, but rather forward simultaneous queries to other search engines and collect the results for you.

Different Tools for Different Jobs

The type of search engine you use depends on what you're searching for. A catalog will return a relatively brief response, whereas an index may provide you with a great deal of information. Thus, catalogs are generally better for searching for general information (e.g., about schizophrenia), whereas indices are better for specifics. If you would like to check the opinions of others about the information you find, search engines that include reviews or ratings are the ones to use.

Search Techniques

Because there is so much information online, you will probably want to refine your searches to filter out irrelevant pages. Understanding how to perform sophisticated searches will save you time and increase your chances of finding what you want. Most search engines let you design and structure your searches in very specific ways, but different search engines have different systems.

Regardless of which search engine you use, it really pays to learn its particular system. For example, how does that particular search engine handle searches that include more than one word? Most search engines will return pages that include any (as opposed to all) of the words. Details are usually accessible via a "Help" or "Search Tips" link. The particular syntax discussed here is that used at AltaVista.

SEARCH TERMS

When searching for multiple words, most search engines by default list first the pages that contain all of those words followed by the pages that contain only some of them, without taking into account the specific locations of the words on the pages. To search for a number of words in a specific order, enclose the phrase in quotation marks.

If a search for a word was too specific, enter just the root of the word immediately followed by an asterisk (with no space between them). For example, enter:

psycho*

to find pages with any variation of psycho: psychotherapy, psychosis, psychopharmacology, and so on.

If search words are capitalized, often search engines will return only pages containing the capitalized words. In many instances it is better to leave words uncapitalized. In that case, search engines will return pages that have the words in either form.

BOOLEAN LOGIC

The use of Boolean logic is perhaps the most powerful search technique. The English mathematician, George Boole, developed an algebra of logic. Boolean

TABLE 1.2
Common Search Techniques

SEARCHING FOR *ATYPICAL ANTIPSYCHOTICS*	EXPLANATION OF SEARCH EXAMPLES
atypical antipsychotics	Pages that contain one or, preferably, both words
atypical AND antipsychotics +atypical +antipsychotics	Pages that contain both words
atypical +antipsychotics	Pages that contain *antipsychotics* and, preferably, *atypical*
+antipsychotics −atypical antipsychotics AND NOT atypical	Pages that contain *antipsychotics* and do not contain *atypical*
"atypical antipsychotics"	Pages that contain *atypical* immediately followed by *antipsychotics*
anti*	Pages that contain any word that starts with *anti*, e.g., *antipsychotics, antidepressants, antisocial, antique*

"operators" are analogous to mathematical operators; they combine basic search criteria rather than basic numerical quantities. These expressions have become the basis for most complex computerized searches. The most common operators are AND, OR, NOT; their symbolic equivalents, "+" and "−"; and parentheses. These simple operators can be enormously helpful when using search engines (see Table 1.2).

To search for pages that contain all of your words, use the capitalized word AND between them. To be interpreted as a Boolean operator, AND may need to be capitalized.

To broaden your search to pages that contain any of your words, use the OR operator between them. This is especially useful with synonyms. For example, searching for:

children OR kids

returns pages that contain either "children" or "kids." Some search engines do not accept the OR operator.

NEAR is a more specific form of the AND operator. It makes sure that both words are not only on the same page, but are located near each other. Simply using the AND operator may not be helpful if the two words are in unrelated sections of a page. Some search engines do not accept the NEAR operator.

Using the NOT operator preceding a word eliminates pages that contain that word. This screens out unwanted information. For example, a search to filter out atypical antipsychotics might read:

antipsychotics AND NOT atypical

Some search engines offer symbolic variations of the Boolean operators AND and NOT. Using a "+" symbol immediately preceding a word (with no space between them) requires that the word be present. Likewise, a "−" symbol immediately preceding a word requires that the word be absent.

These operators are themselves quite powerful but, when used in conjunction with parentheses, they offer even more specific refinement of searches. Parentheses are used in Boolean logic much the way they are in mathematical equations, limiting and ordering relations between variables. The most common use of parentheses is to link two words separated by an OR operator to other criteria using an AND operator. As an example, if you want to find CME programs on panic disorders you can enter:

CME AND (anxiety OR panic)

At times the reverse arrangement may prove better. If you are looking for information on gun control you may want to use:

"gun control" OR (legislation AND gun)

which would return pages either with the phrase *gun control* or with the word *gun* and the word *legislation.*

Some search engines offer limited Boolean logic with radio buttons or pull-down menus. These assist you interactively to work within their limits.

OTHER TARGET ATTRIBUTES

Often, search engines will allow you to limit searches by Web page creation date. This is useful for people who do continuing research on a specific topic, allowing them to limit their results to pages created since their last search.

Some search engines can search specific attributes of a page, most commonly the title and URL. For example, if you are looking for information on herbal medicine and believe that whole Web pages devoted to the subject are likely to have "herbs" in their titles, you could use:

title:herbs

As an example of a URL search, if you are looking for Web pages about psychiatry or psychology, you could use:

url:psych

which would return Web pages that contain "psych" in their URLs and might therefore be expected to (but would not necessarily) be devoted to psychiatry or psychology.

Some search engines allow you to limit your searches to "just the Web" or "just newsgroups." Many search engines provide you with the ability to limit your searches to specific types of media (audio, video, images, etc.).

The Machinations Behind the Magic

It is important to understand that many search engines sell keywords. A pharmaceutical firm can probably purchase search terms like *antidepressant, bipolar,* or *manic-depression* and have a search engine drive traffic to its site. A number of search engines offer certain content first—and designate it "quality" or "recommended"—because they are paid to do so.

Assessing the Accuracy of Information

The sheer volume of information that is available on the Internet is overwhelming. A study done by the NEC Research Institute shows that most people (up to 70%) search on only one keyword or search term (Butler, 2000). This often produces a long list of irrelevant pages.

In addition, virtually everyone with something to sell, a special herb for stress or a new form of meditation, is presenting it on the Web. The "snake oil" salespeople of the previous century have reappeared, and instead of going door to door now have a global reach through this new medium. It is important to know who is running a site and to evaluate their credentials.

Often, large volumes of collected data also contain inconsistencies, errors, and useless data. Schwartz (1993) mentioned two types of inaccuracy: outdated information and inconsistent copies of information. Information often must be timely if it is to be useful. Outdated information often has very little value or, worse, has negative value. And if a search reveals multiple copies of information, how does one determine which version is the accurate one?

A problem confronting the average consumer is how to assess the integrity and accuracy of information presented on the Web. Medical information is offered easily and freely, and it may be difficult for the average reader to understand whether the data presented is factual and whether the writer has the credentials to deliver accurate medical information. Validating information is an important aspect of obtaining information. Information literacy includes evaluating the accuracy of information (which unfortunately further increases the volume of information to be processed by the reader). With the Internet, the person who retrieves a piece of information (rather than the one who publishes it) is most often responsible for determining its accuracy. Because, on the Web, all things are created equal, every user's motto should be "Reader beware."

Future Directions in Online Information

Information access drives information change. Another new element that the World Wide Web has introduced to information transfer is timelessness. The Web is available 24 hours a day, 7 days a week. As more information becomes available, newer information is demanded. The online version of *The New York Times* is updated at approximately 15-minute intervals. People have come to expect that all Web sites, not just those of newspapers, will be up to the minute. This places a tremendous pressure on those sites. While we are sleeping, eating, walking the dog, and so on, they are updating the information they provide.

Distance Learning

In 1899, Kurd Lasswitz, a German philosopher and high school teacher, foresaw distance learning:

> *Not just the telephone [Fernsprecher], but also the television [Fernseher] has been perfected to the extent that one can hear the speaker's words and at the same time also very clearly see his image, his movements, every feature. It is now, of course, no longer necessary to travel a long way to school; teachers and students can gladly stay at home. (Lasswitz, 1899/2000)*

He certainly had the vision to predict the future of online education, but he could not have imagined how popular it would become. The World Wide Web has largely removed the barriers of distance and time.

Technological growth is both necessitating and enabling the evolution of education. According to Chong (1997), the rapid rate of innovation has had a threefold impact on information:

- The volume of information is growing at a spectacular pace.
- The information is becoming increasingly specialized and complex.
- The life expectancy of information is shortening.

At the same time, technological innovations have had a tremendous impact on our ability to make information available. There is a broad consensus that jobs in this information age require lifelong education (Hall, 1996). More and more, people are seeing themselves as perpetual students. Textbooks are no longer able keep up with the rapid change of information. Distance learning and the new "virtual universities" open up doors that were previously closed.

Digital Health Records

What types of online information lie ahead? After many years of inventing different brands of wheels, information technology is finally heading toward standardization and integration. That convergence will be based on the Internet. Since its inception, communication on the Internet has been governed by specific protocols. Those standards are now among the most accepted for the transmission of electronic information, and the Internet is therefore the most viable basic structure on which to build information systems that can be widely adopted.

Technologists and administrators see Web-enabled "digital health records" or "electronic medical records" as the holy grail of health care information systems. Having that infrastructure built on a single platform—the Web—will save the health care industry hundreds of millions of dollars every year.

Using the Web, clinicians will have instantaneous access to all of the usual elements of the paper health record in addition to several novel ones. Only electronic media can offer error checking, formulary status, insurance information, coding guidelines, integration of laboratory results, consultations, other patient data, and links to the latest clinical and pharmacological studies.

Patients will interact easily and freely with their own digital health records and their physicians. This will empower consumers and enhance patient–doctor communication. Many patients want to manage more of their own health care, and with the Web they will be able to do so.

XML

HTML, the language of the Web, is being revised and upgraded. Currently, it is a very simple language with a limited number of commands, and it merely tells the browser how to display the information on the page.

How, then, to find that information is also an issue. The finding of information usually has not been a consideration for authors and has only been an afterthought for publishers. In order to make online information even more accessible, salient sections could be labeled or marked and then referred or hyperlinked to directly.

An example of this might be a Web page on depression that contains sections on depression in children and adolescents, depression in the elderly, etc. In order to find the individual sections with search engines, each section would need to be marked with an appropriate tag.

This is a minor example of what potentially could be a very complex process. It would be up to authors and publishers early in the process to identify and mark smaller bits of information that are important.

An evolving language that could enable this is extensible markup language (XML). XML allows information not just to be displayed, but also to be labeled with tags or "metadata." With XML, tags can let a reader (or a search engine) know, for example, what kind of information is being presented (a scientific paper, a news story, or an advertisement), when it was produced, who the author is, and where the author is located. Specialized tags can also represent fields in a database, thus allowing readers to interface with them. Tags are even being developed that allow readers to add their own tags.

Personalization

We will see more Web sites that "learn the user." Customizable Web interfaces will allow readers to indicate their preferences; for example, to select particular types of news, articles, or journals. Web sites are beginning to remember the interests of users and to offer suggestions accordingly.

Information Overload

Finally, as our wealth of information increases, so does our need for better tools to manage it. We are facing an overabundance of data. Carlos Fuentes, as quoted in Wurman (1989) noted that "the greatest crisis facing modern civilization is going to be how to transform information into structured knowledge" (p. 194). We need to study the different ways in which people look for and use information. We need to make information easier to find. Better information retrieval systems will benefit everyone.

Conclusion

The Internet has become the most important communication medium since the telephone. The everyday workplace relies on computer networks. Workgroups electronically share projects as well as gossip. The World Wide Web is pulling the world together. Computer connections are enhancing human connections. Over the millennia, as humans traveled the Earth, they developed relationships with other cultures and races. The distances between people became shorter, the ties between them firmer. Our global computer network is now connecting millions of people who never would have connected in any other way. The world has truly become smaller and more accessible.

> *There is no practical obstacle whatever now to the creation of an efficient index to all human knowledge, ideas and achievements, to the creation, that is, of a complete planetary memory for all mankind....*
>
> *The whole human memory can be, and probably in a short time will be, made accessible to every individual. And what is also of very great importance in this uncertain world where destruction becomes continually more frequent and unpredictable, is this, that ... it need not be concentrated in any one single place. It need not be vulnerable as a human head or a human heart is vulnerable. It can be reproduced exactly and fully, in Peru, China, Iceland, Central Africa or wherever else.... It can have at once, the concentration of a craniate animal and the diffused vitality of an amoeba.*

Those are the words of H. G. Wells. If only he knew how prophetic his words were. He published these words back in 1938 (1971 p. 86–87) before the existence of the computer, let alone the Internet.

References

Baur, C., & Deering, M. J. (2000). Proposed frameworks to improve the quality of health web sites: Review. *Medscape General Medicine, 2*(5) [Online]. Available: www.medscape.com/viewarticle/418842

Boswell, J. (1987). *Life of Johnson* (R. W. Chapman, Ed.). Oxford: Oxford University Press. (Original work published 1791)

Butler, D. (2000). Souped-up search engines. *Nature, 405,* 112–115.

Chong, N. S. T. (1997, July). *Higher education over the Internet: Dawn of the virtual university.* Paper presented at the UNESCO Regional Conference for Higher Education, Tokyo.

Editor's Introduction to Vannevar Bush's "As We May Think." (1945, July). *Atlantic Monthly, 176*(1), 101–108.

Fine, S. F. (1982). Human factors and human consequences: Opening commentary. In A. Kent & T. J. Galvin (Eds.), *Information technology: Critical choices for library decision-makers* (pp. 209–224). New York: Marcel Dekker.

Hall, P. (1996, July). *Globalization and the world cities.* Tokyo: United Nations University/Institute of Advanced Studies. (Working Paper No. 12)

Horton, F. (1983). Information literacy vs. computer literacy. *Bulletin of the American Society for Information Science, 9*(4), 14–16.

Hubbard, S. (1987). *Information skills for an information society: A review of research* (ERIC Digest). Syracuse, NY: ERIC Clearinghouse on Information Resources. (ERIC Identifier ED327216)

Lasswitz, K. (2000). *The distance learning school* (K.-E. Tallmo, Trans.) [Online]. Available: art-bin.com/art/ofernschule_e.html (Original work published 1899)

Murray, H., Jr. (1996, March 8). *Methods for satisfying the needs of the scientist and the engineer for scientific and technical communication* [press release]. Washington, DC: Author.

Pew Internet & American Life Project. (2000). *The online health care revolution: How the Web helps Americans take better care of themselves* [Online]. Available: www.pewinternet.org/reports/pdfs/PIP_Health_Report.pdf

Pool, R. (1994, October 7). Turning an info glut into a library. *Science, 266*(5182), 20–22.

Russell, B. (1948). *Human knowledge: Its scope and limits.* New York: Simon & Schuster.

Schwartz, M. F. (1993). Internet resource discovery at the University of Colorado. *IEEE Computer, 26*(9), 25–35.

Warren, B., Kramer, T., Hyler, S. E., & Kennedy, R. (1997). Using the Internet. In L. J. Dickstein, M. B. Riba, et al. (Eds.), *American psychiatric press review of psychiatry* (Vol. 16, pp. VI-49–VI-67). Washington, DC: American Psychiatric Press, Inc.

Wells, H. G. (1971). *World Brain.* Freeport, NY: Books for Libraries. (Original work published 1938)

Wurman, R. S. (1989). *Information anxiety.* New York: Doubleday.

2

The Internet "Expert": Promise and Perils

Ronald Pies

QUESTION

HEY DOC, THANKS for being there! PLEASE PLEASE PLEASE answer my question!!! I'm soooo depressed! St. John's Wort hasn't done anything for me, and I'm finally desperate enough to try a *real* antidepressant. Which one do you recommend? Thanx!!!

QUESTION

Dear Doctor, I am an attorney with your malpractice insurance company. We have recently become aware of your Ask the Expert service for Mental Health InfoSource. Please respond at your earliest convenience to the following questions so that we may clarify the extent of the applicability of your current policy with us.

1. Do you consider this activity part of your medical practice? Do you limit it to states in which you possess a current license?
2. How do you know if someone is telling the truth? Might they not be distorting, or even fabricating, the "facts" of the case?
3. What if someone is suicidal, sends you a question, and then kills himself or herself after you respond—or do not respond?
4. What if you don't know the answer to a question?
5. What if you're wrong?
6. Have you ever been sued or threatened with a lawsuit for answering—or not answering—a question?

Thank you for your prompt attention to this matter.

QUESTION

Pies, you SOB! A patient of mine sends you a question, and you, without even meeting, let alone examining, her, tell her I gave her the wrong medication! She filed a complaint against me, and I had to get a lawyer. And they don't come cheap! Plus I don't get the big bucks from Harvard like you do. Sure, sit up there in your ivory tower and give us peons down here in the trenches a hard time. I hope you have good malpractice insurance, I'm not going down alone!

As the putative expert at the Mental Health InfoSource "Ask the Expert" site (mhsource.com/expert), I have had to deal with hundreds of challenging questions from both professionals and consumers. Fortunately, the examples just shown have *not* been among them. However, these three hypothetical queries do raise a number of important issues I have thought about quite a bit. But before delving into these matters, it might be useful to provide a little background material.

For the past 5 years or so, I have been answering questions posted online at mhsource.com. Each week, the webmaster, Ms. Heather Orey, selects about six questions, originating from both professional and nonprofessional users. The site has a fairly detailed disclaimer, which I will discuss later. Over the years, questions have ranged from "Dear Abby" type queries ("I just broke up with my boyfriend and I feel terrible! What should I do?") to arcane questions about vagal nerve stimulation or dopamine receptors. Overall, most of the questions are reasonable attempts to obtain appropriate professional information, often to supplement what the questioner has learned from his or her health care providers.

The three bogus questions at the beginning of this chapter are another matter. The first presents the consumer or online user—please note I do not use the term *patient*, because that carries specific medical-legal implications—who seems to be in desperate need of advice. This individual wants a specific medical recommendation—in this case, a particular antidepressant—and sounds as if he or she may need one. It is always tempting in such cases to "take the bait," but I try never to do so. It is one thing to provide general information about a specific medication, such as its usual side effects or its on- and off-label indications; it's quite another to recommend that someone actually use that agent. One response represents medical education; the other, arguably, represents inappropriate medical practice.

I have argued elsewhere (Pies, 1998) that prescribing medications over the Internet—in the absence of an examination of the patient—is medically (if not legally) inappropriate. The same holds for any specific medical recommendations other than those I call *heuristic*. These are recommendations that lead to further knowledge or provide the questioner with an appropriate therapeutic environment in which to resolve the problem. In contrast, *proscriptive* recommendations are those that deliberately limit or cut off a questioner's options, for example, "You have to stop taking medication X immediately" or "You should stop seeing Dr. Y right away." Similarly, *prescriptive* recommendations are specific positive interventions aimed at a presumed disorder or condition, for example, "You should be taking twice as much Prozac as you are now taking" or "You need to undergo immediate ECT for your depression." I try very hard to avoid both proscriptive and prescriptive responses. Heuristic responses usually take the form of "You should strongly consider seeing a psychotherapist so that your problem may be more thoroughly evaluated" or "You might want to discuss medication Z with your doctor." I believe these heuristic responses really amount to medical education. They say, in effect, "Your problem is the type that ordinarily requires more scrutiny and thought." This is quite different than providing a questioner with a diagnosis and recommending a course of treatment.

There are exceptions, of course. Sometimes I do dispense what I would call commonsense generic advice of the sort one's mother (or father) might provide, for example, "Eat a healthy, balanced diet" or "Make sure you get adequate sleep." Even such seemingly innocuous advice has its risks in certain circumstances, however. For example, telling a patient to get plenty of exercise may sound like common sense, but it could be harmful if the online questioner has serious cardiac problems. (Instead, I might say, "Exercise would be a good idea if your family physician approves.") There is another instance in which I do offer prescriptive advice: when a life may hang in the balance. Despite the disclaimer we have on our site (more on that later), some users insist on writing in a state of crisis, for example, "I'm about to blow my head off. The gun is cocked at my side. I'm so depressed. What do you recommend?" In these unfortunate circumstances, I have no real choice except to advise them to get to an emergency room as soon as possible. (In a sense, this advice is both prescriptive and heuristic.)

This brings us to some of the medical-legal issues raised by the (fortunately fictitious) attorney for my malpractice insurance company. Clearly, I do *not* consider the responses I provide online to constitute a part of my medical practice. Rather, in my view, this activity falls under the scope of medical education, similar to writing a column in a newspaper on, say, "How to Improve Your Mental Outlook." Thus, from my perspective, there is no issue of state medical licensure involved, any more than there would be if a newspaper article I wrote in Massachusetts were also published in California. An even more apt analogy might be a psychiatrist's giving a response to an anonymous questioner in the audience after a lecture on, for instance, depression. I believe that as long as such a response is educational and heuristic in the sense I have indicated, there is no practice of medicine involved. As to how I know that someone is "telling the truth" online, the answer is that of course I don't. But that is no less true when I see a patient in my office—after all, we know that patients with Munchausen's syndrome fabricate all sorts of claims, as do those with sociopathic traits. Regarding suicidal individuals, I'm sure it's no surprise that I worry about these people. At the same time, I do not believe that I have set up any expectations, much less any contractual understanding, that I am available as an online "crisis manager" or "emergency room doc." This gets us into the disclaimer that is prominently displayed on the Web site. To summarize, the disclaimer states that

> Owing to time constraints and the volume of mail, our expert is unable to reply to every question submitted. Ask the Expert is intended solely as an informational service, not as a substitute for routine or urgent medical evaluation, treatment or consultation. . . . Our expert's suggestions should not be construed as medical opinions aimed at establishing a diagnosis or course of treatment. Diagnosis and treatment are complex and require comprehensive face-to-face assessment over long periods of time. Individuals under active treatment should not construe information contained in this column as replacing or superseding recommendations of their clinicians. Rather, information in this column may serve as a point of discussion between patients and their individual clinicians. Similarly, clinicians should appreciate that suggestions made in this column, without benefit of direct assessment, are not intended as direct consultative recommendations. . . .

As for being wrong, I'm quite sure that has happened. But doctors may be wrong in any setting, whether in the office, the journal article, or the lecture hall. The issue here is what are the consequences of my being wrong? If questioners are appropriately referred for further evaluation, and if both proscriptive and prescriptive responses are avoided, there should be no serious adverse consequences for the questioner if my response turns out to be wrong. And finally, no, I've never been sued or threatened with a lawsuit for giving, or not giving, an answer to a question. But I also never take that for granted! Incidentally, various freelance writers' unions provide "media perils" insurance policies designed to protect nonphysician writers who may offer advice on a variety of subjects.

The third fictitious question does raise a troubling issue, although not one I have had to deal with as yet: how to avoid antagonizing or circumventing the online questioner's primary care physician or psychiatrist. There is one simple rule I always try to follow: avoid telling someone that what his or her doctor is doing is wrong. This applies specifically to medications, recommended procedures, or diagnostic conclusions. On the other hand, even this rule has its exceptions: If a patient wrote in saying, "My doctor says I need to have sex with him each time we meet in his office. Is this wrong?" my answer would be a loud and clear "Yes!" I also provide generic "educational" information that might lead a perceptive consumer/patient to raise certain pointed questions with his or her primary care physician. For example, a patient writes, "My doctor has been prescribing high doses of barbiturates for my depression. This medicine hasn't done me any good. In fact, I think I'm worse. Is what my doctor is doing wrong?" In that case, I might reply in very general terms, along these lines: "There is no evidence I know of showing that barbiturates are helpful for treating depression. In fact, there is evidence to the contrary. It would be prudent to discuss your doctor's rationale for using barbiturates in your case. It may be that he or she has a convincing explanation. On the other hand, it might be wise to ask him or her to arrange for a psychiatric second opinion so that you can get appropriate expert advice regarding your medication." Now, it might be argued that this response is merely diplomacy, and that, in effect, I have called this person's doctor an imbecile. But my response *does* allow for the possibility that the doctor has a "convincing explanation"; thus, it avoids accusing him or her of any wrongdoing. My advice also remains heuristic, and does not instruct the patient to stop taking the barbiturates.

In the next section, I provide some actual questions from the mhsource.com Web site (edited, in some cases, for conciseness and clarity), followed by my responses. I then provide, in light of the principles I have just discussed, some commentary on my replies.

Examples from Ask the Expert

What Would Happen if He Stopped Taking the Medication?

QUESTION
Joe is 47 and has had 2 weeks of not sleeping—some nights no sleep, others 2 or 3 hours. He was worried about doing well at work. This culminated in his first visit to a psychiatrist. After being given Ambien, he still did not sleep the next night. His psychiatrist put him in the mental ward of the hospital for a week, where he went on Zyprexa and Zoloft. He was sleeping well and felt much better. This continued for about 3 weeks. Then he had a period of 5 days when he had less sleep and drank more coffee than usual. He started worrying and ruminating about things and now has feelings of worthlessness, loneliness,

no energy or desire to do things; wants to sleep; and even has thoughts of suicide. He's scared he won't get better, because it's been about 3 months since all this started. Joe keeps wondering if part of the problem is the medication he's taking and what would happen if he stopped taking it. I wonder if the caffeine might have caused him to relapse. Also, what would you suggest if he doesn't improve on these medications? He has had his thyroid tested and the blood work, but has not had a CAT scan or MRI.

ANSWER
This sounds like a very difficult situation not only for Joe, but also for you. First off: Although I can't directly advise you on Joe's diagnosis or treatment, I would caution any patient with Joe's symptoms against stopping medications without the treating physician's approval. The symptoms you describe—feelings of worthlessness, no energy, thoughts of suicide, and so on—must be taken very seriously, and sound very much like a major depressive episode. That Joe's doctor prescribed an antipsychotic medication—Zyprexa—also suggests that the doctor thought Joe was having some psychotic symptoms, such as delusions or hallucinations. I can't say if that was an accurate assessment, but I can tell you that psychotic symptoms can often accompany a severe major depression. (By the way, caffeine is rarely the cause of these kinds of symptoms, although in rare cases, very high doses of caffeine can worsen manic or psychotic symptoms and certainly can lead to insomnia.)

Stopping antidepressant and antipsychotic medication could put a patient with Joe's symptoms in great danger. If the medications are not working or are producing troublesome side effects, then the patient needs to sit down immediately with the psychiatrist and figure out a new approach. This certainly could involve the use of different medications or—even more effective for psychotic depression—electroconvulsive therapy (ECT). (For more information on ECT, see related material on this Web site.) Some alternative medications Joe could discuss with his doctor include risperidone, quetiapine, or clozapine (all antipsychotics); and venlafaxine (an antidepressant). The fact that Joe had a good response to Zoloft and Zyprexa at first suggests that his doctor was on the right track, but it never hurts to get a second opinion from another experienced psychiatrist. Ideally, this should be discussed with the primary physician and not be an "end run" around his or her authority. A medical school department of psychiatry would be a good source of referrals. Given Joe's age (over 40) and lack of personal or family psychiatric history, it would certainly be important to rule out neurological or underlying medical causes for his symptoms. Many psychiatrists (myself included) do order imaging studies of the brain (such as an MRI) for first-onset episodes of major depression in this sort of case. Three months may seem like an eternity when you are suffering, but it's not all that unusual for cases of severe major depression to require 3 or 4 months to resolve fully. Most depressed patients do eventually get well, and I hope things do work out well for Joe soon.

COMMENTARY

My main goals in responding to this question were as follows:

1. To provide useful, general information without telling the questioner (the patient's wife?) what should or should not be done.
2. To introduce the idea that suddenly stopping antidepressant or antipsychotic medication is often a bad move, but not actually telling the questioner "Joe should not stop" these medications; hence, the generic formulation, "Stopping antidepressant and antipsychotic medication could put a patient with Joe's symptoms in great danger."
3. To encourage Joe to discuss his problems with his prescribing psychiatrist.
4. To suggest that a second opinion might be a good idea *without* suggesting that this be done "behind the back" of Joe's psychiatrist.
5. To provide the questioner with alternative diagnostic and treatment strategies that could be discussed with Joe and *with Joe's doctor.*
6. To leave the questioner with a sense of hope and a more reasonable perspective on the course of major depression. (I did not provide a diagnosis for Joe, although I did say that his symptoms "sound very much like a major depressive episode.")

In short, I tried to provide a heuristic, rather than a prescriptive or proscriptive, response.

What Tools Exist for Self-Analysis?

QUESTION

What tools exist for self-analysis? How can I assess whether or not I have a mental health problem?

ANSWER

I'm all in favor of self-knowledge, but I'm not a big fan of self-analysis—or self-diagnosis. I believe there are too many pitfalls for so-called consumers. It's easy to persuade yourself that there's "really nothing serious going on with me" when an objective professional observer would see that, indeed, there is something *very* serious going on. *In short, the way to assess whether or not you have a mental health problem is to see a mental health professional for an evaluation.* If you are having trouble affording an appointment, try getting in touch with the local chapter of the National Alliance for the Mentally Ill (NAMI). Their hotline is 1-800-950-NAMI. NAMI is very good at helping people gain access to mental health care. Having now given you the official line, I will point out that New York University has quite a good Web site that offers a variety of screening tests on depression, anxiety, and other psychiatric disorders. The authors are careful to point out that a given test "does not replace in any way a formal psychiatric evaluation. It is designed to give a preliminary idea about the presence of mild to moderate depressive symptoms that indicate the need for an evaluation by a psychiatrist." The Web site is at www.med.nyu.edu/psych/public.html. It also has useful information on advocacy groups, articles, books, and so on. But seriously—mental health evaluation is not a "take-home kit." Please do see a psychiatrist, psychologist, psychiatric social worker, or other mental health professional.

COMMENTARY
Imagine how any mental health professional would feel if he or she found out that a consumer filled out some sort of self-test questionnaire on the advice of the professional; concluded that he or she had no problem; and subsequently wound up in a serious, life-threatening major depressive bout. Imagine the medical-legal repercussions if that consumer or his or her family were to accuse the online expert of having contributed to the missed diagnosis by pointing the consumer toward the self-test! This, clearly, was the scenario I wanted to avert, and I went out of my way to provide another heuristic recommendation: to obtain a complete mental health evaluation. At the same time, I did not want to appear totally unresponsive to the question, and thus provided the address of the NYU Web site along with that site's own caveat.

I Have a Patient Who Is Interested in Using Hypericum

QUESTION
I am a registered general nurse and an aromatherapist, and I have a patient who is interested in using hypericum as a treatment for mild depression, but is naturally anxious about any interactions with other drugs she is taking. Clearly, she needs to discuss this with her GP, but if she were able to take relevant, up-to-date information with her this would help her GP. The drugs she is currently taking are bendrofluazide, thyroxine, atenolol, phylopidine, and cerivostatin. If any of your research has shown any problems when hypericum is taken with any of these drugs, I should be most grateful if you could let

me know as soon as possible. In general, would you advise against over-the-counter remedies like hypericum unless the patient first consults with his or her doctor?

ANSWER
To answer the last part of your question, yes, absolutely, I would advise against over-the-counter (OTC) or herbal remedies like hypericum (St. John's Wort) unless the patient first consults with his or her doctor!

The simple truth is this: we do not know how hypericum or most other herbs/OTC products interact with the vast majority of prescribed medications. "Up-to-date" information is really limited to published case reports, usually of adverse events—I know of very little *prospective* research in which specific OTC remedies are being investigated in combination with prescribed medication.

Numerous interactions with hypericum have been reported, however (*PDR for Herbal Medicines*, 2000). For example, hypericum may have adverse interactions with selective serotonin reuptake inhibitors, cyclosporine, protease inhibitors, Coumadin, oral contraceptives, theophylline, and digoxin. In addition, concomitant use with other photosensitizers, such as tetracyclines, sulfonamides, thiazides, and quinolones, is not recommended. I could not find any published articles on interactions between hypericum and bendrofluazide, atenolol, or thyroxine, *but the absence of such reports is no guarantee that hypericum may be used safely with these agents.* I could not find the terms "cerivostatin" or "phylopidine" in my database—sorry, perhaps these are drugs specific to your country? As a general rule, hypericum tends to affect agents metabolized via the CYP 3A4 enzyme system. Hypericum appears to induce (increase the activity of) 3A4, thereby reducing blood levels of agents that are metabolized by 3A4. This can result in, for example, reduced levels of digoxin. For more details on herb–drug interactions, also see the article by Fugh-Berman in the January 2000 *Lancet.* The bottom line: Using over-the-counter and herbal remedies is always a bit of a gamble, particularly when combined with other pharmaceuticals.

COMMENTARY
I'm not quite sure what an aromatherapist is, but I tried to address this questioner as a colleague. Indeed, he or she seemed to be fairly sophisticated, recognizing at least the possibility that hypericum might interact with prescribed medications—a realization that has escaped some psychiatrists. I tried to provide this practitioner with some up-to-date information without being overly (and inappropriately) reassuring. Instead, I provided the questioner with a reference that provides much more detailed information.

Do You Think This Could Be a Case of Amnesia?

QUESTION
In a case where a woman is present at the stabbing deaths of her children and is stabbed herself, but says that she woke up to find this situation, do you think this could be a case of traumatic or psychogenic amnesia? Do you think it could be accurately diagnosed in 12 sessions with a psychiatrist, and do you think that standard psychological tests would be required for the diagnosis? Another question is, if her memories of what happened in the minutes after she "awoke" seemed to change in detail but not in substance, would you consider this to be a psychological thing or would you consider her to be lying?

ANSWER
You are raising some of the most vexing and controversial questions in all of psychiatry. The whole range of issues covering repressed memory, traumatic memory, implanted memory, and malingering continues to provoke heated debate even among knowledgeable mental health professionals. Without commenting specifically on the case you raise, I would make a number of general points:

1. Some recovered memories of trauma probably *do* correspond to actual experiences (see Brewin & Andrews, December 1998, *Clinical Psychology Reviews*).
2. Nevertheless, to quote one expert in the area: "Hypnosis and other methodologies employed in psychotherapy may be beneficial in working through memories of trauma, but *they may also distort memories* or alter a subject's evaluation of their veracity" (italics added).
3. Use of projective tests, such as the Rorschach, may be useful in distinguishing authentic from false memories of trauma (Leavitt & Labott, July 1996, *Journal of Traumatic Stress*).
4. On the other hand, the "either-or" dichotomy between "recovered" versus "false" memories may be misleading. Some researchers believe that *in the very same patient, both false memories and traumatic amnesia may coexist* (Baars & McGovern, March 1995, *Consciousness and Cognition*). Baars and McGovern believe that trauma victims differ in how suggestible they are and how likely they are to dissociate in the presence of a trauma (e.g., seeing someone killed or actually killing someone). This means they may differ as to how easily their memories can be modified or manipulated by others, as well as how much they are able to compartmentalize traumatic memories into areas of their mind not accessible to conscious recollection. There are scales that can help assess suggestibility and

tendency to dissociate (e.g., the Dissociative Experiences Scale). There are also scales (such as the "F" scale on the Minnesota Multiphasic Personality Inventory) that help point to malingering or exaggeration of symptoms. However, there is no single test that can infallibly distinguish false from authentic memories. In the sort of complex case you discuss, I believe that skilled evaluation by an *expert in traumatic memory* is critical. Inexperienced therapists or evaluators may inadvertently suggest things that become a part of the person's memory even though these things did not actually occur. On the other hand, regarding slight changes in the details a patient may recover as evidence of "lying" would be unwarranted. The bottom line: It is sometimes impossible to tease out what really happened from distortions of the patient's memories. The truth must be approached from the standpoint of *all* the evidence, including psychological, forensic, and that obtained through specialized techniques such as hypnosis. I think you will find much more of interest in the articles I've cited.

COMMENTARY

I could practically feel the subpoena in my hands after reading this question! This sort of question is, to borrow a phrase from gestalt therapist Fritz Perls, a "bear-trapper." The putative "expert"—by providing *specific opinions relevant to a specific case*—could easily be providing an opportunistic attorney, plaintiff, or defendant with ammunition he or she could use in court. That expert, so far as I know, could easily be compelled to appear in court, having offered such specific conclusions. Thus, my response was predicated on the phrase, "without commenting specifically on the case you raise." I then went on to make some very general points about recovered memories, followed by the heuristic suggestion that "skilled evaluation by an *expert in traumatic memory* is critical" in such cases. The kind of answers provided are consistent with the Web site's stipulation that answers are "informational" in nature, not prescriptive.

I Have No Attachment to My Young Son

QUESTION

I have a big problem: I have no attachment to my young son. What I mean is, I feel nothing toward him. I know this sounds bad, and I've sent him to live with his father. I have two daughters and love then both dearly, but I know something is wrong when it comes to my son. I know I love him, but some days when people ask how many children I have, I have to stop and think. I have been struggling with this feeling since before he was born, and I think

I'm going crazy. Am I wrong to think that something is wrong? I want to know if this is a disorder or if there is something wrong with me.

ANSWER
What you describe does not sound crazy, but it is clearly very distressing to you. I think you are right to be concerned about your relationship with your son, but I can't tell you if you are suffering from a particular disorder. It does seem clear, however, from what you say, that you are a person who can feel great love for your children. It's not that you are a cold, emotionless person— but something seems to have *blocked* you from feeling toward your son the kind of affection you have for your daughters. Of course, I can't tell you why that block is there. For some women, it might be that the birth of the child occurred under adverse circumstances, for example, the mother might not have wished to become pregnant, but felt that she had no choice. For other women, it might be a matter of having conflicts related to men, so that a son might symbolize something quite different than would a daughter. Some women become quite depressed after the birth of a child (less commonly, before the birth). If the depression is not treated and resolved, it could affect the mother's ability to feel emotionally close to the child. Whether any of these scenarios fits with you, of course, I can't say. But I do urge you to seek some counseling on this important issue. It would also be prudent to have a complete physical exam to make sure there is no medical problem that could be contributing to the way you are reacting. Then I would suggest seeing a psychotherapist with special expertise in family therapy or women's problems. With some time and work, I believe you can understand the nature of this problem and feel better.

COMMENTARY
Here was a questioner in obvious pain and distress. Does she have a mental disorder? Is she "crazy"? Of course, there is simply no way any clinician could answer such questions without a full, face-to-face evaluation. (I suspect the *unasked* question was, "Am I a bad mother?") Thus, the dilemma for the online expert is to provide an empathic and *realistically reassuring* response without foreclosing diagnosis and possibly treatment.

Every Day I Regret Not Succeeding When I Attempted Suicide

QUESTION
Last fall, I attempted suicide. My husband is having a hard time coming to terms with my severe depression. We have tried marital counseling, and I am currently seeing a therapist once a week and a psychiatrist once a month.

Nothing has improved, though, and every day I regret not succeeding last fall. I know I shouldn't think this way, but it can't be helped. What should I do?

ANSWER

You are suffering so much right now, you understandably think it "can't be helped"—but it can. It sounds to me as if your depression has not responded adequately to treatment. This can occur in as many as 20% of cases of major depression and is usually called "refractory" or "treatment-resistant" depression. You do not discuss what medications, if any, you are now taking or have taken, but I doubt very much that you have been tried on all the available (and very effective) options. It also strikes me that once-a-week therapy may not be sufficient for you right now, as suggested by the fact that you are writing to me. It is possible that more frequent meetings would be of help or that you require psychotherapy of a different kind. Two kinds that can be very effective for depression are cognitive behavioral therapy (CBT) and interpersonal therapy (IPT). If you are not involved in either one of these, you may want to ask your therapist about them. (Even if your therapist does not provide CBT or IPT, you might benefit from a group that does use one of these approaches.)

You should also discuss medication. I am assuming that your psychiatrist is prescribing something for you now, but that it hasn't worked. There are dozens of other things that might help, including newer agents like Remeron or Effexor. And while you may have a lot of negative feelings about ECT (electroconvulsive therapy), it is a safe, highly effective, and often life-saving treatment for treatment-resistant depression. You owe it to yourself and your family to consider and explore *all* the available options before concluding that things are hopeless. I also encourage you to contact the National Depressive and Manic Depressive Association (NDMDA) for information about support groups for patients and their families. Call them at 800-826-3632 or try their Web site (www.ndmda.org). You may also call the Samaritans at any time, day or night, and speak anonymously with a counselor (dial your local information number). I know it is hard for you to believe this, but depression can be surmounted—and I urge you not to give up!

COMMENTARY

The temptation to tell this questioner what she "should" do is probably great for many of us with extensive experience treating depressed patients. However, I tried to resist this, while indicating to the questioner that her current treatment "may not be sufficient"—the key here is "*may* not be." Readers will doubtless notice that I *do* use the word *should*—but I do so only in the heuristic sense of "you should also discuss medication" options with the psychiatrist. I provide some alternative sources of help for this questioner—the NDMDA and the Samaritans—but not sources that are likely to *interfere* with the questioner's current caregivers. To be sure, this is a judgment call—some psychiatrists might not want their depressed patients to contact the NDMDA—but this was a risk that I felt was worth taking.

Conclusions

Serving as the online "expert" for a mental health Web site is, on the face of it, an act of some hubris. After all, who among us is really an expert on all facets of mental health care? From time to time, I consult with my own private cadre of "experts," particularly when the question is outside my clinical experience. I sometimes suggest that the questioner contact various experts in the field and provide a mailing address. (I don't give out individuals' phone numbers.) I also recommend books or reference materials that I have personally read or that originate from organizations (such as the American Psychiatric Association) that I know and trust. Sometimes, I suggest that a questioner "might be interested in reading" a book that I personally have not read, but know about, based on a literature or online search. I avoid using the term *recommend* in such cases.

Despite the caveats presented on the Web site and within my own responses, it is always possible that some individuals will misuse the site; for example, writing in the midst of a psychiatric emergency or substituting a suggestion I make for the specific recommendation of their own physician. But this hazard is present whenever an identified "authority" speaks to the general public, whether on the television, the radio, or the Web. For example, I have great respect for Dr. Timothy Johnson's medical advice, as provided on ABC television. Dr. Johnson is usually very circumspect in his "recommendations" and goes out of his way to avoid circumventing the authority of the questioner's doctor, but he can't prevent a listener from using bad judgment, and neither can I. There is a legal presumption, in our society, that people are competent until proven otherwise. I govern myself online by this presumption even though, in any given instance, I might be wrong.

Providing educational material online has been a challenging but rewarding activity for me. It is quite different from meeting with a patient in my office, and I try to convey this fact in the Web site disclaimer. Although the benefits of online education may be limited, the breadth of the Internet is virtually unlimited. I like the idea of assisting hundreds, perhaps thousands, of people at a time. At least that's my hope. I have received a number of very gratifying responses to some of my online replies, and—so far—only one negative comment. (The latter was related to my favorable remarks on ECT and originated from a consumer advocate who was rather misinformed about the risks of ECT.) One maxim I try to keep in mind at all times is that of the great physician and philosopher Maimonides: "Teach thy tongue to say, 'I do not know,' and thou shalt progress."

References

Baars, B. J., & McGovern, K. (1995, March). Steps toward healing: False memories and traumagenic amnesia may coexist in vulnerable populations. *Consciousness and Cognition, 4*(1), 68–74.

Brewin, C. R., & Andrews, B. (1998, December). Recovered memories of trauma: Phenomenology and cognitive mechanisms. *Clinical Psychology Reviews, 18*(8), 949–970.

Fugh-Berman, A. (2000, January 8). Herb-drug interactions. *Lancet, 355*(9198), 134–138.

Leavitt, R., & Labott, S. M. (1996, July). Authenticity of recovered sexual abuse memories: A Rorschach study. *Journal of Traumatic Stress, 9*(3), 483–496.

Physician's Desk Reference for Herbal Medicines (2nd ed). (2000). Montvale, NJ: Medical Economics.

Pies, R. (1998). Cyber-medicine [letter]. *New England Journal of Medicine, 339*, 638–639.

I would like to thank Heather Orey, the Webmaster at mhsource.com, for her assistance and good judgment over the years.

3

Using E-Mail to Support the Outpatient Treatment of Anorexia Nervosa

Joel Yager

CLINICIANS AND patients are e-mailing one another at increasing rates. Quasi-diagnoses, consultative advice, and sometimes prescriptions have been provided over the Internet through sites such as AmericasDoctor (www. americasdoctor.com); CyberDocs (www.cyberdocs.com), "where the doctor is always in"; and WebMD (www.WebMD.com), where one can "pay an office visit to the future of health care." Working analogously to urgent care physicians, most of these clinicians do not establish ongoing relationships with their patients. Many offer medical guidance on an "as needed" or "call-in" basis, filling the perceived gaps that result from the fact that many patients desire more contact with and explanation from their physicians than they usually receive during office visits.

Conversely, clinicians increasingly e-mail their own patients. One recent survey conduced by the Healtheon Corporation reported that of 10,000 physicians who were sampled, about 85% used the Internet and about one third exchanged e-mail messages with patients (Stroh, 1999).

Youths are the most avid e-mail users. Not only adolescents and young adults but even latency-age children now routinely have e-mail access at home or in school. A growing number of junior and senior high schools and most colleges provide e-mail accounts for all of their students, and adolescents increasingly also have private e-mail accounts. Adolescents find e-mail to be a powerful means of communication. Some reportedly spend hours on the telephone, but sometimes hang up to "talk" instead via e-mail about particularly sensitive matters, finding it easier, perhaps less embarrassing, to communicate about highly personal or gossipy issues through this newly cool medium of text. Telephone communications might convey more emotion than the youths care to share, and therefore give them less control. Studies suggest that e-mail may give greater voice to those who are less dominant in organizations and relationships, and may provide opportunities for the emergence of other aspects of the self than ordinarily appear in face-to-face meetings (Kiesler, Siegel, & McGuire, 1984; Turkel, 1984, 1995). Physicians working for online companies such as those mentioned earlier have also sensed that some patients have less trouble asking or talking about embarrassing health-related issues via e-mail than in face-to-face encounters.

These observations suggest that systematically incorporating e-mail contacts into ongoing treatment relationships in psychiatry and other fields of medicine may afford benefits to some patients. A few early uses of e-mail have been described in several modes of Internet-based psychotherapy (Murphy & Mitchell, 1998), crisis counseling (Wilson & Lester, 1998), and support groups (Dunham et al., 1998). This chapter describes the evolution of my use of e-mail into a routine adjunctive method in the treatment of outpatients with anorexia nervosa, some of my cases, and some of the issues that arise when e-mail is made part of a practice. I've now incorporated e-mail in one way or another into the treatment of about 15 outpatients I've seen for anorexia nervosa. The benefits of using e-mail in a large percentage of these cases have become evident to me. It helps with many but not all patients. However, using e-mail in a practice occasionally leads to complications, and their management requires specific sensitivities. As well, several issues related to professional "netiquette" and ethics merit discussion.

The Evolution of My Use of E-Mail

I started using e-mail with patients more than a decade ago, to handle simple administrative tasks such as scheduling appointments, processing requests for prescription refills, and arranging for laboratory tests. To enhance my and my office's ability to communicate as efficiently as possible, I began to routinely ask patients for their e-mail addresses and provide them with my own. Initially, only a small percentage of patients had e-mail. Over the decade, the number has increased to the point where it's now rare for patients not to have e-mail. Patients who were traveling or who had moved out of the area would send e-mail messages to ask specific questions or, increasingly as time went on, to let me know how they were doing. Some occasionally wrote longer, detailed e-mail messages filled with reflections and emotion. My responses were usually brief. Depending on the tone of the message, however, I sometimes felt it was indicated to arrange to speak with the patient over the phone, sometimes for an extended session. When I moved from Los Angeles to New Mexico 5 years ago, several patients asked if they could maintain our contact and correspond with me via e-mail, and I've had enduring relationships with some of my former patients in this manner.

Since moving to New Mexico, my thoughts about the clinical utility of e-mail have expanded. In part, this coincides with the fact that the majority of my patients, especially the adolescents and young adults, now have e-mail. In addition, by virtue of my practice, I've been required to consult with and sometimes offer ongoing services not only to patients who live nearby in Albuquerque, but also to some who live in remote areas, from 70 to several hundred miles away, and who cannot easily come in for frequent office visits. E-mail has also been a godsend for communicating with some of the busy providers who are also involved with these patients; e-mail is more convenient for some communications than is the phone. As my work with e-mail has evolved, it's become clear to me that this technology may be particularly useful to clinicians in the management of outpatients with anorexia nervosa. The following case material illustrates how I've used e-mail with patients whom I've treated myself in regularly scheduled office-based therapy and those about whom I've been consulted for second opinions or ongoing assistance with treatment.

Examples of the Adjunctive Use of E-Mail

E-Mail to Enhance Weekly Sessions

In this situation, e-mail was used several times a week to supplement weekly to every-other-week office sessions for psychotherapy and medication management. A, a 17-year-old high school senior, had had anorexia nervosa for 3 to 4 years. This 5'4" young woman had been training as a runner since age 8. Menarche occurred when she was $12\frac{1}{2}$, but that had been her only menstrual period. She weighed about 110 pounds at that time, her highest weight ever. That same month, during the course of a gymnastics meet, her coach offhandedly mentioned that she could afford to lose 5 pounds, which prompted her to cut all fat-containing foods from her diet. Several other personal and family stressors occurred simultaneously. She lost 15 pounds. By age 16, A's weight had fallen to 88 pounds. She was hospitalized on a medical unit for 2 weeks by her family physician, who intubated and tube-fed her and discharged her at a weight of 93 pounds. At that time, she started working with a psychologist and started to take paroxetine 40 mg/day, prescribed by her family physician. Her weight was up to 100 pounds when I first saw her, about 9 months later.

She described herself as "stuck" and unable to go higher. She had not menstruated since that one occasion at age $12\frac{1}{2}$. Her food choices were markedly restricted—she ate snacks but no real meals—and she was exercising about 1 to 2 hours/day. She estimated her caloric intake at 500 to 700 calories/day at its lowest, but thought that on rare occasions it increased to 1,700 calories/day. She felt that her thighs were still too big, but she was very unhappy about having very small breasts. She purged rarely (perhaps twice via self-induced vomiting in the 6 months prior to consultation, and not at all for many months prior to that) and used no laxatives, diet pills, or illicit drugs. A compulsive organizer to a fault, she saw herself as perfectionistic, ritualistic, and orderly, doing the same things in the same way every day. However, it was uncertain whether any of these symptoms were present prior to her anorexia nervosa. She complained of ongoing symptoms of depression—she felt worthless, lonely, empty, and indecisive, and was anxious and irritable with her family regarding food issues.

When I first met A and her parents, it was clear that she needed a big push to make headway, but she was avoidant and reluctant. Neither A nor her parents would even consider a hospital program. A was able to agree, intellectually, that some weight gain was necessary to allow her to achieve a physiological endpoint at which menstruation and ovulation would occur. She also noted that she had stopped growing at age $12\frac{1}{2}$, was much smaller than her siblings and parents, and harbored the hope that she might be able to gain height. The program we devised included weekly to every-other-week outpatient therapy for A, family visits with A and her mother every 2 to 3 weeks, a lot of reading material on eating disorders for A and her family, elimination of active exercise, a 2000- to 2500-calorie diet together with visits with the registered dietician with whom she'd been working, bone densiometry, continuing medications, and frequent e-mail messages between sessions to focus on the amount and variety of her meals. Looming behind this plan was the explicit threat, supported by her parents, that if she didn't make adequate progress within 2 months she would have to stop school, be hospitalized in an eating disorders program, and interrupt her senior year in high school.

WEEK 1

A was able to eat about 2,100 calories one day but only about 1,750 calories on other days. She agreed to weighings, but asked her dietician not to tell her the weights at this point. She was obsessed with the upcoming Thanksgiving holiday, which her family was sharing with friends, regarding what she would be able to eat, count the calories of, and control. We discussed and started homework exercises based on cognitive therapy principles. She also started to describe recent highly emotive family arguments—concerning her relationships with her father and older sister and their relationship with one another—that were disturbing to her. Her mother was distraught, feeling caught in the middle. These severe family tensions were the focus of several sessions with A alone, her mother alone, and the two of them together, until strategies were devised that successfully defused the crisis and permitted the family to move on.

> Hi Dr. Yager-meister! How are you today? I'm doing ok. I'm feeling confident that I can do this. Today I have had no diet soda yet and don't plan on drinking any. I am going to eat a p-nut butter and pita sandwich instead of a light bread sandwich. I'm going to buy myself a regular yogurt and eat a total of 1900 calories total. I'm a little nervous but also positive that I can do this. A

WEEK 2

We focused on monitoring, cognitive appraisals, and deconstructing firmly held beliefs. She talked about her academic life; she appreciated the fact, intellectually, that overcoming the anorexia nervosa would help her to adapt and contend with college and life in the big city. E-mail reports came several times a week describing meals, estimating caloric intakes, and occasionally mentioning issues at home or in school. She reported a few small milestones: being able to eat meals with friends and family, expanding her food repertoire with small bites of forbidden things, adding chocolate candy snacks and cookies into her meal plan.

> Hey Dr. Y! Happy Thanksgiving—too bad the vacation's over. I had a bad Thanksgiving day.... I got very uncomfortable and anxious at the place we went and I ended up going home. I felt horrible but got over it. I'll tell you about it on Thursday.... Thanks for typing back.... Oh yeah, I had a package of p-nut M&Ms on Saturday. WAHOO! Later! A

> Today I plan to eat 2200 but God! I don't know what else to add. I feel like I'm eating all the time and I'm not eating anything light at all! Oh well.... I was thinking about having some M&Ms again today cuz they're easy and yummy calories! We'll see. I gotta run. Have a happy day. A

WEEK 6

Dr. Yager, Hi there sir. How are you today? I'm ok. Not great. Yesterday in gym I was wearing an outfit that I haven't worn in a while.... It's always been smaller than my others, but it felt different. I started thinking about and noticing my body more. It sucked. I can tell my butt is bigger, and I feel like my thighs are humongous. They look gross to me when I look down at them. My stomach and waist feel different too. I feel gross, I mean when I pay attention to my actual body. Physically I feel good—energetically and all. I'm a little sick with a cold, but other than that I'm ok. I feel awkward and a little sad about stuff, mostly my body and boys.... I just felt kinda blah last night and a little today too. Maybe it's PMS ... a freaky thing for me to think about! Maybe I just need to get back into the swing of things.... I don't know. Thanx for reading (listening sorta). I'll talk to you more on Thursday. Bye-bye. A

Hi A. I'm glad to be able to comfort you. You're really on the right track, and "slumps happen." See you tomorrow. JY

Hi Dr. Y. Thanx for your comforting response. I still feel pretty icky, but I'm eating the right amount of calories anyway. I'm just in a slump, but that's how things go: up and down, up and down. I'll see you tomorrow. A

WEEK 8

Her weight had been increasing and was now about 108. We were dealing with continuing unhappiness with large thighs, family matters, the fact that she received few social invitations from either girl or boy classmates, and uncertainty about college.

Hey Dr. Dude. Sorry I didn't get to e-mail you yesterday. Things are ok. I'm not terrible, but I'm not great ... I'm just kinda here. My hormones must be kicking in hard core because I've got zits all over my forehead! I don't really have much to tell you. Oh well.... Talk to ya later. A

Hey! Congratulations on the zits—that's a great sign, having to do with the return of hormones and health. They'll clear up OK. I'm sending you lots of good encouragement. I know you're "just there" for now—things will definitely have an upswing. Take care and keep up the good work. See you next week. JY

WEEK 12

One of our goals for her was to be able to eat pizza. As with many patients, pizza had taken on huge import—because it's both an important social food and obviously contains various fats.

I had a very nice day. I ate a piece of pizza with my mom, but it was reallllly big so I cut some of it off. I estimated about 400 calories for it. It was good but I felt incredibly full after eating it. I'm still alive though. . . . A

WEEK 17
About 114 pounds.

I don't know what my deal is with calories again. I just feel fine where I am. I gained the weight you wanted me to gain, and now I don't want to move on. It's weird. I just feel scared of calories. It's silly I know. I'm worried about colleges and decision-making too. I just feel blah. I have a terrible case of spring fever too. AHHHHHHH! I have no motivation. Oh well. See you tomorrow. A

WEEK 18
Her weight was about 115 pounds.

YUCK!!!!!!! I HAD A PERIOD!!!!! I CAN'T BELIEVE I'M WRITING THIS TO YOU IN AN E-MAIL. IT'S DISGUSTING!!!!! Talk with ya later, dude! A

WEEK 22
Her weight hovered around 116 pounds; she was eating about 1,700 calories/day and exercising very little. She had been accepted at the prestigious Ivy League school of her choice. Her acne calmed down, her hormones were in full bloom, she had another period, and she was pining for a boyfriend. We defined as a goal the ability to eat normally so that no boy she dated would ever think she had any weirdness about food.

Great news! You'll never guess what happened last night! Well, you might guess, but I'm not going to give you a chance. I called John. . . . We decided to make plans to get together. He suggested we get a bite to eat. Perfect, huh? We went to Ragin' Shrimp and I ordered gumbo. I ate the shrimp and some of the vegetables and was full! I would've preferred to eat what he got (or something like it) rather than the gumbo . . . more seafood and less other stuff, but oh well, next time! We sat and talked til about 11 or so! It was really great. We both want to go out again too! Yay! I'm really happy and proud of myself for the dinner thing! Have a great weekend! Take care. Bye for now. A :)

Hi A. I'm so happy to hear this. Our discussion yesterday [concerning the fact that she was now sending out different "messages" regarding availability and interest in boys, as well as the need for her to eat socially in such a manner that her dates wouldn't suspect that she had an eating disorder] was perfectly timed, wasn't it! You just keep it up. Cheers, and have a great weekend. JY

WEEK 23

Hi. I saw [my dietitian] yesterday. I've gained 1 pound since the last time I saw her. I'm a little weirded out about this because I've been doing fewer calories. However, it is only one pound. Anyway, she and I compromised and I'm going to work my way up slowly. I'm doing 1700–1800 this week cuz in the last six months I gained 10 lbs. really fast . . . the fastest I ever have. I'm scared and want to slow down a little. Does this sound ok? Later! A

I realized that she was starting to come within range of a healthy weight.

Hi. You're really doing well, and remember: keep your eye on the big picture, and the big goal. The only way to get there is to keep moving in that direction. Best wishes, JY

WEEK 24

Hi. Things are fabulous! I'm totally enchanted and haven't been obsessing about food. I haven't told John anything about my eating disorder . . . maybe in a while . . . if it's the right time. I'm feeling great! I'm soooo happy cuz of John. Later dude! A

WEEK 25

She graduated from high school, threw a class party at her home, and celebrated by eating some of the cake she and her mother had ordered.

Hi A. Congratulations on graduating! Consider yourself hugged. JY

Her mother, to whom she showed this note, loved it. After graduation and before her departure for college, we continued to see each other every week or two. At this point, away from her private school e-mail account and having to share an e-mail address with the rest of the family, e-mail traffic slowed down. She maintained her clinical improvement. She still struggled with increasing her food choices, but was making progress.

WEEK 28

We'd been working on expanding her food choices so that her eating in groups or on dates wouldn't seem unusual.

Hi! Yesterday I went to the store and bought a box of ice cream sandwiches! Not low-fat or light or anything . . . the real things! Today I had a "Chug-a-lug" chocolate milk! It was yummy. I've also had mashed potatoes. I've been eating all this good stuff that's new. . . . The only bad thing about these new foods is that I am sure to know the calories I'm taking in :(I'm trying to get my calories up and am slowly getting there. . . . Later dude. A

PATIENT'S SUMMARY AND EVALUATION

E-mail focused on daily eating. Outcomes included a weight gain of 15 pounds and reasonably good biopsychosocial recovery. Here is A's own assessment regarding the use of e-mail in her treatment (provided via e-mail, of course):

> Pros: It's great for keeping me in check with things . . . you know, incentive to do well! It's nice to hear back from you. . . . It makes me feel like I'm more than just a once-a-week patient. Reading responses is encouraging. It's a good way to release what's on my mind at the moment that I might otherwise forget to mention in a session, a good way to stop what I'm doing and take a minute to reflect on how well I'm taking care of myself. Of all the things I HAVE to do in the day, it's the (or one of the) best things to HAVE to do.

> Cons: It's one more thing to have to do! Reporting bad news because of my own doing! Forgetting to check in regularly makes me feel bad :(

Then, contrasting her use of e-mail from her private school account and at home:

> It's a pain to log on to my dad's e-mail. I don't have my own private account at home. . . . Others can ("but don't") read my mail. Re: the privacy thing, my dad has access to these messages, but he says he doesn't ever read them. I believe him, but would rather keep things vague as you did in your previous message. By the way, thank you for your abstractness. . . . For that one message, my dad opened it and sat here while I read it. "But he usually doesn't read them." I'm sure he was just being courteous and opening it for me cuz I was right here, but you never know. . . . I was actually a bit scared that he would read a response that wasn't abstract. Thank you again!

E-Mail to Monitor Treatment From a Distance

B was an 18-year-old girl, scheduled to start college at the end of the month I first saw her. Her primary care physician was concerned about her alarming weight loss over the previous 2 years.

Prior to the onset of her eating disorder, B described herself, and was described by her concerned parents, as completely well in all respects, perhaps a bit perfectionistic. During her junior year in high school, at a height of 5'2", her weight fell from 98 pounds, her previous highest weight, to 82 pounds. By the time I first saw her, nearly 2 years after the onset of her eating disorder, she weighed 77 pounds. She acknowledged, intellectually, that she was too thin. She denied overexercising, binge-eating, purging, the use of illicit substances, obsessions or compulsions not related to food, or mood disturbances. Although her parents' style of relating entailed considerable bickering, family boundaries toward B and her sister were appropriate and the family was basically loving and supportive.

B resented being dragged in by her parents to see me. She felt coerced. During our initial meeting B tried to disguise her emaciation with baggy overalls and a sweatshirt and acted in a charming, pseudomature manner, but cried easily, especially on hearing her parents express how upset they were about her situation. She tried to minimize her food restrictions relative to her parents' account of her behaviors. At least intellectually, she was able to say that she should weigh 95 to 100 pounds. She also acknowledged her inability to eat enough to make this happen.

Although I immediately raised the option of a hospital program, she and her parents all strongly requested a trial of outpatient care that would permit her to start school. After consulting with student health physicians, her primary care physician, her nutritionist, and a psychotherapist who would see her weekly, I agreed to set up a "short leash," closely monitored outpatient treatment trial to permit her to start school. We set a minimum goal of weight gain of 1 pound a week. A detailed meal plan was established. She wrote out and signed an explicit written agreement to the effect that if she were not able to make this weight gain during the semester, she and her parents would agree to a leave of absence from school and she would enter an inpatient hospital program. She also knew that if her weight fell below 77 pounds during the semester she would have to interrupt school to be hospitalized immediately. B was to be seen at least weekly by a student-health physician and the psychotherapist. She received no medication. I was to take on the role of "overseer," with some sort of contact at least every other week. B signed permission forms so that all involved health care providers could share information. During the course of assessment and treatment, I frequently communicated via e-mail with her student-health physician, nutritionist, and therapist. Her parents also got into the loop, e-mailing us reports of her weekends at home and other issues, with B's knowledge. When corresponding about her with other providers, to protect her confidentiality in the event that someone else saw those messages (an unlikely but nevertheless possible occurrence), I never used her full name. Because I was to see her in person only intermittently and infrequently, I asked her to e-mail me weekly concerning her activities, her eating, and her progress.

B began the program highly motivated and with enthusiasm, ate meals and snacks on a regular schedule, and gained about 3 pounds within 2 to 3 weeks. Here are extracts from our e-mail communications:

WEEK 4 OF THE SEMESTER

Hello! In a continuation of our communication, I wanted to let you know that my weight was up again, to 81 lbs. I'm sure you know that I spoke with [my nutritionist] and have a new eating plan, the one we decided on together. I had a long talk with [my student-health physician] today to let her in on the new plan. However, in the future I am not sure that I will need to spend a lot of time speaking with her as I will be seeing [my therapist] and speaking with [my nutritionist], and in a comment [my student-health physician] had made earlier in the year she said that it wasn't fair to me to take a long time at each visit, but [I should just] get my weight checked and speak with her as needed. I think my mother e-mailed you regarding this as well. . . . Thank you again for your time, and I will be in touch! B

But progress was difficult.

WEEK 6

Dr. Yager, The latest update is not as good as I would have liked—I was down 1 lb., which cancels the weight gain I had last week. I think I was retaining water, which put on the added weight. I was disappointed, but now am more determined than ever to make this week bring the most weight gain I can possibly have. Other than that disappointment I am doing well, and really having fun in my classes. Some of my teachers are really good, and I just am so interested in the new things I am learning! Plus, I am meeting new people STILL and becoming closer to the friends I already had. Well, have a great week, and thank you for your time! B

Hi, B. Although it may be something of a pain, I'd strongly urge you to keep a personal calendar to go over with me or [your nutritionist] or [your therapist], recording exactly how many of the food items in the plan you actually eat each day—to record the number, portion size, amount finished, etc., so that you can calculate realistic caloric intakes, and discuss any specific problems you may have with the plan. Best wishes. JY

B followed the instructions. A few days later, she wrote:

Dr. Yager, I have been keeping a diary of total calories at every meal/snack, which includes what I have eaten and how much (i.e., portion size), but I can be more specific as the diary just has the numbers. Also, when I get home I can fax the addendum to you. Have a nice weekend! B

And 3 days later:

Dr. Yager, I just received your note regarding keeping track of HOW MUCH I eat—I will definitely do that, though I have been doing that all along. Also, to let you know, the meal plan must be working because I have gained another pound. The addendum should reach you today, as I left it with my parents to fax. Thanks for your time, and talk to you soon! B

WEEK 8

Dr. Yager, Just wanted to check in with you for this week. Today I was 83 lbs., which is once again a 1-lb. gain. Yeah!! Have a good week and talk to you soon. Thank you for your time. B

WEEK 9

Dr. Yager, Great news! I have gained 3 lbs. and am now up to 86 lbs.! I am slightly apprehensive though. . . . I am keeping in mind however how both you and [my primary care physician] said that there will be some large and small weight increases, and the more important thing is to look at the big picture. But things are continuing in the right direction! B

Dear B, Again, good for you!! The big picture is exactly correct. There WILL be bigger and smaller shifts. . . . Stay with it! JY

WEEK 11

Dr. Yager, Today I weighed in at 86 lbs., (again, but when I looked at the last few weeks, it averages to 1 lb. a week). Have a great Thanksgiving! B

Hi, B. You have a great Thanksgiving too. As long as you maintain the one pound per week increase you're headed in the right direction. I suggest that you keep a calendar and enter the weight numbers each week so that you can graph your progress—it's a good mental trick! Best to your family. JY

WEEK 12

Dr. Yager, Hello! I hope you had a nice holiday. Today I weighed 86.5 lbs. Another piece of information that is positive is that although I have not had a period yet, I have started spotting, which tells me that my body wants to have a cycle, but still needs more weight to go through with it. Have a good week! B

B, Once again, you're going in the right direction. Keep it up, and keep in touch. JY

WEEK 13

Dr. Yager, Today I weighed in at 87.5 lbs. Another gain!! Yeah!! Have a great week and thank you for your time! B

That's GREAT! You're doing something right, aren't you. Best wishes, and keep in touch. JY

My next contact with B was 6 weeks later. She called me to update her status and to "tell you the good news." Her last weight, a few weeks prior, had been

92 pounds. "I'm not sure what it is, but over the Christmas break everything fell into place." Her family was delighted and supportive. She was still working closely with her therapist, feeling more alert and energetic, and able to take on activities at school that she couldn't the previous semester.

At a 2-year followup B's weight was 100–101 pounds. She'd been having normal periods for at least 7 to 8 months. This was the important indicator for her. Aside from cheese, she was eating everything and said that she "learned to use food rather than have food use me." She'd started weightlifting, "not like a body builder," and that had helped her to gain weight. Her only other exercise was "a little bit of running." School was going well—she was getting straight As—and she was considering medical school or neuroscience. She reflected that she was somewhat "antisocial" when she started school, which she attributed to being malnourished and anorexic, but that in the past year she'd blossomed and now had as much of a social life as she could handle. B attributed her recovery largely to her therapist and to her own desire to get well. She worked with her therapist intensively, about twice a week, for about 4 to 5 months, and also included her parents in the sessions occasionally. After that, she felt that "I didn't have anything more to talk about."

PATIENT'S SUMMARY AND EVALUATION
B considered e-mail a "once-a-week sign-in," but didn't think it played much of a role in her recovery. She resented having to check in. Her e-mailed assessment:

> In that respect, it made me feel I had to check in with someone, made me feel younger; it didn't matter if it was e-mail or phone or face-to-face. When I came to you, you had the upper hand. I felt fear, anger, resentment. Come to think of it, given that you made me check in, e-mail was a good way to be in touch, since it provided some distance. I think e-mail can be effective when a person is on their way to recovery. It's quick and so easy just to keep in touch.

E-Mail to Monitor Food Intake Daily

I was asked to see C, a 50-year-old social worker, by her psychologist, an eating disorders specialist, who had been following her for the binge-eating/purging type of anorexia. C had had a mild eating disorder in college and graduate school, but had maintained herself at a healthy weight with only slight food preoccupations until her mid-40s. At that time, she encountered new job-related stresses and began eating excessively, including binge-eating a lot of easily accessible fatty foods, so that her weight, usually between 130 and 140 pounds at a height of 5'6", ballooned up to almost 240 pounds over a period of a year and a half. At that point, she was diagnosed with hypertension and hypercholesterolemia and was told that she absolutely had to lose weight. She approached her diet with a vengeance, eliminating all fats and adopting an entirely vegetarian diet that was deficient in protein, allowing less than 20 grams/day. For months, she also binged on sweets several times a week, and on these occasions purged by self-induced vomiting. She lost weight rapidly, going down to 110 pounds, started to become easily fatigued, and experienced excessive daytime sleepiness, forgetfulness, and intermittent confusion. Recognizing that she needed help but refusing to consider hospitalization, she started outpatient care with a psychologist who was knowledgeable about eating disorders. The psychologist started a program of cognitive-behavioral therapy designed to increase C's caloric intake and food choices, but the patient remained very reluctant to eat more or differently. At that point I was asked to consult.

Over a period of three months, I saw C three times in the office (the first two visits for detailed assessment and treatment planning), but I maintained nearly daily e-mail contact with her as part of the plan. Her other treatment consisted of weekly visits with her psychologist. She took no psychiatric medication. After extensive laboratory testing, elaborate analysis of her diet, and clear demonstration that her protein intake was inadequate and her fat intake was negligible, I gave her explicit goals for increased calorie and protein intake (she still could not bring herself to take in more than a small amount of fat), asked her to e-mail me a daily account of her meals, and requested that she include an daily analysis of the amount of carbohydrate, protein, and fat. After initial protest, C gradually increased her intake to 40 or more grams of protein and between 1,700 and 1,800 calories a day, and very slowly increased her fat intake. Some illustrative exchanges follow.

Dear Dr. Yager, If I told you that I WOULDN'T be surprised at all about my fat and protein intake, would I still have to calculate it? No fat, except for what is naturally in food, is the way I lost all my weight in the first place. It's not as if I'm not already obsessed to death with what I'm eating and the weight gain that it will no doubt cause by trying to put this stuff back into my diet. If I need to do this, by the time you see me next Thursday I will be a stark, raving, non-functioning lunatic. So, you had better have a straightjacket handy and maybe some Valium. I assure you I am not overreacting. C

Hi C. I certainly don't mean to make you feel worse, so only do what you can really do at this point without driving yourself crazy. My goal is not to torture you—of course. However, if you're not going to be able to modify your diet and regain your health on your own, we'll have to talk about what other assists exist. See you next week. Take care, and be well! JY

I also instructed her to take two fish oil concentrate capsules a day—for her "brain"—and as a way of starting to desensitize her to adding some fat to her diet.

$\frac{1}{2}$ cup red beans = 117 cal, 7 g protein, 0 g fat
1 cup strawberries = 45 cal, 0.9 g protein, 0.6 g fat
$3\frac{1}{2}$ oz mango = 67 cal, 0.8 g protein, 0.3 g fat
1 pkg grits = 100 cal, 3 g protein, 0 g fat
7 oz baked potato = 220 cal, 4.7 g protein, 0.2 g fat
2 tbsp unpopped popcorn = 100 cal, 0 g protein, 1 g fat
1 tbsp veg oil = 120 cal, 0 protein, 14 g fat
1 pretzel without butter = 470 cal, 11 g protein, 0.5 fat
4 oz sugar-free, nonfat frozen yogurt = 56–68 cal, 3.28 g protein, 0.24 g fat

Dr. Yager, I bought the book you told me to get and I also got those "horse pills" you told me to take two of. I can't believe I'm actually swallowing fish oil. At 2000 mg a day I might get fins and it seems like I wouldn't have to worry about eating any other fats in my diet either. C

Great work on the protein. Now you need to work on the calories, too, so that your body doesn't simply break down the protein to use for fuel since there's not enough carbohydrate around. We want the protein to be available to replenish lost stores and to get your brain on track again. Cheers! JY

A day or two later, she wrote:

Dr. Yager, Nothing is up except that my body felt like it had to ease up a little bit. Starting tomorrow I will be doing better. I bought the wrong beans and didn't notice it until too late. . . . I would eat more right now except that the beans are way too filling and I couldn't possibly hold it. Also, it's too late to eat. I just need a little time. I can't be perfect overnight. I really will do better starting tomorrow. C

Hi C. I'm glad to hear that you think you'll be able to do better. Please take some encouragement, and please don't deceive yourself (or us), either, about what's realistic for you to be able to do on your own. AND please keep posting me about your intake as you've been doing. Stay in touch. JY

During 3 months of contact, we achieved the initial goal of increasing her protein intake. Her symptoms of sleepiness, sluggishness, and confusion improved significantly. We are still working on increasing her dietary fat.

PATIENT'S SUMMARY AND EVALUATION

C's assessment of the utility of e-mail in her care (provided via e-mail, of course) was quite positive:

> To tell you the truth, I hate it. But I realize that this was the price I had to pay not to go into the hospital. I really value being an honest person—so I knew I couldn't lie to you. By having to write down all the calories and protein every day I had to really confront what I was doing. You really made me face it every single day. Without the e-mail, I would have ignored my eating—let it slide—but having to write every day I couldn't ignore it.
>
> E-mailing back and forth every day with a progress report is a real good thing for the part of me that wants to get well and healthy. Having to give a daily report on everything I eat encourages me eat to the way I'm supposed to because it makes me aware of what I'm eating and what I need to eat, such as more protein, etc. E-mailing also gives me a sense of security because there is always an open door between me and someone who is there to help me if I need it. Getting feedback on how I am doing is also very encouraging (or can be frightening). For the part of me that still wants to lose weight, having to report what I eat each day is a real pain. This part of me feels pressured into eating when and what I don't want and it makes me feel crazy because I always have to think about it. Now that I've told the secrets of the way I think, I guess I'll be e-mailing for the rest of my life. (NOT!!!)

E-Mail to Transition Between Care Providers

D was a 22-year-old woman recovering from severe anorexia nervosa. Her weight had dropped from 125 to 67 pounds 3 years earlier. Although it had increased to 115 pounds since then, she had significant residual psychiatric symptoms. I was asked to see D when the psychiatrist with whom she had been working—and who had prescribed several medications for her—was about to leave the area. The new psychiatrist D planned to see wasn't going to be available for a few months. I was to provide care during the interim and serve as an ongoing consultant after she started with her new psychiatrist. We met in my office on four occasions, about a week to two weeks apart; I also met once with the patient and her mother and once separately with her mother. D told me that she used e-mail and felt comfortable with using it to write about her progress and to ask questions, so I also had her e-mail me frequently to let me know how she was doing.

The transition went smoothly, and we continued to have frequent e-mail contact until she became well connected with her new psychiatrist, with whom, with her consent, I shared her e-mail messages. In addition to giving me details about specific eating and mood disorder issues and answering my medication-related queries regarding side effects, D also e-mailed me about a big argument her parents had that resulted in their decision to separate and divorce, her reactions to various health care providers, and social and vocational developments in her life. Her mood improved to some extent, and her diet and weight were both maintained.

PATIENT'S SUMMARY AND EVALUATION

The first thing that pops into my head is that e-mail makes communication between doctor and patient much better because you can "talk" on a far more consistent basis. Instead of seeing your doctor only once a week, or even just twice a month, you can be in daily contact. I know that especially when I was at my worst and seeing my [original] psychiatrist only once or twice a month, I didn't do [what I was supposed to] as much as I should have. Then, when it would be closer to seeing him, I'd actually do [those] things because I didn't want to lie to him—I could say I did do some things, sometimes, at least. It seems like people with eating disorders want so badly to please their doctors (just as they want to please everybody). I felt good when my doctor was proud of me, since for so long everybody felt very annoyed with me, and I felt so much shame within myself for all the problems that MY problem caused my friends and family. Mostly it's just a feeling . . . you feel proud. If I was talking to my doctor more, I would have felt like that much more often. Trying to change a person with an eating disorder is a hard, long, and difficult thing, and encouragement is so important. Another common trait is having such low self-esteem. Just feeling like somebody cares enough about you to get to know you and takes time out of their extremely busy schedule to e-mail you on a pretty much daily basis gives that poor self-esteem a lift. . . . It really does feel good.

Another thing with me, I don't know how many people with eating disorders feel this way, but it's hard to trust somebody when you've put so much effort into doing what you think will make you happy. Keeping my feelings and thoughts to myself was the safest and only thing I could do. Through e-mail that trust could possibly grow faster cuz you get to know your doctor better, since you have so much contact. I know I went on and on, but my fingers just wouldn't stop typing. I hope it makes some sense, I'm not all that good at getting across what I'm trying to say. Thanks for asking, I hope I gave you a decent answer.

E-Mail to Communicate With Family Members

E was an 11-year-old girl who developed anorexia nervosa 9 months before I saw her. She had developed marked obsessions and was jumping rope compulsively. At the time of consultation, her height was $4'8\frac{1}{2}''$ and she weighed

53 pounds; her weight had been as low as 50 pounds but, hoping to avoid hospitalization, she was trying hard to increase her caloric intake. However, every meal, every bite, was an occasion for great obsessing, and she was exhausting her mother, who was trying valiantly to help E to eat.

It seemed clear to me that E would require hospitalization in a specialized eating disorders program. I agreed to help the family find a program and, until then, to consult with E's managing pediatrician and the family regarding her day-to-day care and to try to find a qualified local therapist with whom E and her family could work several times a week. E agreed to e-mail me her daily intake. Over the next few days, E wrote a few e-mail messages, plaintive notes saying how hard it was for her to eat and how much she hoped that she would not have to be removed from her family to be hospitalized. Over the ensuing week, however, she actually lost 2 more pounds, so hospitalization became inevitable. Here are some communications with the family. As you can see, communication was mostly with P, her father, a high-tech scientist, in part because he used e-mail constantly at the office and was trying to handle administrative aspects of the treatment. Our e-mails dealt much more practically with issues of placement and insurance coverage than e-mails with patients usually do. Excerpts follow:

> Dear P, I'm still trying to locate therapists who might be on your plan and who have good reputations and skills in dealing with eating disorders in young adolescents. I noted that you wrote that [one doctor] might be available—she's actually quite experienced in this area and is excellent with children from what I know. I'll get back to you as soon as I hear anything. Please tell E that I received her e-mail and I really appreciate how hard she's trying and how hard this is—please tell her from me to keep up all of her good efforts and to hang in there. Please give my best to E and to your wife. JY

The following morning, I communicated with E's pediatrician right after E had a scheduled office visit with her. E had lost 2 more pounds and clearly needed more intensive treatment. Her pediatrician arranged to have E hospitalized at a local community hospital, pending probable transfer to a university-based eating disorders program out of state. That morning I wrote:

> Dear P, I understand from [her pediatrician] that E lost another 2 pounds—I think that you and your wife have done what you can to deal with E at home and that at this point hospitalization is really necessary. You and your wife shouldn't see this as any shortcoming on your part—I can assure you that E has a very serious problem and that it merits very serious care. I understand from [her pediatrician] that she's going to have E hospitalized at [the local hospital] under the care of [another doctor] pending probable transfer to the eating disorder program at [the out-of-state hospital]. You can anticipate that E is going to plead, cry, tug at your heartstrings in all sorts of ways, etc., to keep from being hospitalized. Please realize that as much as it hurts you to see her suffer, hospitalization at this point is most

likely essential for her physical safety. She's been losing weight at too rapid a pace for safety. I understand that the decision for hospitalization will be reviewed by a medical board. You (and your attorneys) should be aware that two recent court decisions, one by an appellate court, ruled that medical insurance coverage to deal with the malnutrition of anorexia nervosa should be at the same level as coverage for medical conditions. . . . Please let me know what transpires. If you think it might help, I'd be happy to see the two of you again—you can call my office for an appointment. Good luck! JY

We had crossed e-mails. At about that time, I received the following e-mail from P:

Dr. Yager. I just received a phone call from my wife. E has lost an additional two pounds and is being taken directly to [the local hospital]. I spoke to our mental health plan today. This was before I heard this news. The plan representative suggested that they do a doctor-to-doctor consultation between you and a doctor from their staff to get E prequalified for an inpatient plan should that become necessary. It is becoming more and more clear to us that it will be. I have provided your phone and e-mail address to the plan for the consultation. I hope this was ok. The good news is that under our current plan we do have what appears to be fairly good inpatient program coverage. I know that the [out-of-state hospital] program is considered an in-plan facility. I have asked that they search for other facilities in the NM, TX, AZ, UT, and CA areas. . . In any event, as we discussed in your office, my wife and I are committed to getting E the treatment she needs to deal with this condition. I am leaving for the hospital as soon as I finish this e-mail. I assume [her pediatrician] will communicate with you. Thank you for your help. P

P and I exchanged several e-mails over the next few days concerning administrative issues, such as:

Dr. Yager, I got both of your replies and I appreciate your comments about our insurance. Hopefully it won't become necessary. Surprisingly E seemed to want to go to the day program at [the local hospital]. I think this is in part because she knows the next alternative is the out-of-state inpatient program and in part because she realizes she needs help she has not been getting. She has really been wanting someone she can work with on a regular and frequent basis who can help her through this problem. The therapist that we dealt with at [the local hospital] last night indicated she would set a weight below which E can't drop (or else she would recommend hospitalization in a medical unit) and will work with E over the next few days to determine whether she thinks they can deal with E as an outpatient at [the local hospital] or if inpatient treatment is required. While we are somewhat skeptical due to the fact E is the only one of eleven kids at [the local hospital] who has an eating disorder, the therapist does seem to have some experience in dealing with eating disorders. E also seems to like her. My wife and I are going on the assumption we will be going to an inpatient program as soon as we can get in, but in the meantime E has expressed a strong desire to try and make this program work. In any event, it seems to be providing some additional motivation to get calories in the short run. I spoke with our mental health plan representative again today. . . . P

E-Mail to Co-Manage a Patient

F was a 23-year-old patient who developed anorexia nervosa with binge-eating and purging at about age 15. By the age of 22, when she returned to her parents' home after being unable to successfully remain in college in another state, she had advanced osteoporosis. Because she lived more than 100 miles from my office in Albuquerque, coming for office visits on a regular basis proved very difficult for her, especially because she was ambivalent about coming for treatment in the first place. She felt that her parents, successful ranchers, were coercing her to get treatment, using their financial support as leverage. She resisted efforts at treatment by dragging her feet about making appointments, often missing scheduled appointments (including visits with her primary care physician in her own town) and refusing to carry out assignments. F felt that she had to conquer her illness on her own, but she was making little progress in doing so.

We met in my office a few times for a full and frank discussion of her perspectives on her eating disorder and life in general. She was exceptionally bright, charming, informed, and self-deluding, and insisted that she would have to do her treatment entirely on her own if it were to mean something to her. After her initial general medical workup, she refused to schedule followup blood tests, in part because she fainted whenever she had blood drawn (a classic vasovagal reaction). Although she initially agreed to e-mail how she was doing regarding her eating and symptoms, she was slow to do so and managed to send only a handful of e-mails over several months. Finally, she failed to respond to either e-mail or phone contacts. Over the months, I received a number of distressed e-mails from her parents and also from M, her primary care physician. Using e-mail, I was able to collaborate with M on her management:

> Dear Joel, I need your advice. I saw F again after quite some time. Her weight is down to $95\frac{1}{2}$, initially $93\frac{1}{2}$, maximum 99. She admits she eats only one meal a day, although says she isn't binge-eating. She says she has had two

periods, although one was very slight. She feels good physically and is very happy with her school and a boyfriend whom she likes very much. She plans to return to school and is working this summer. However, she was upset and said she wants to meet again in several weeks to get weighed; she will try harder and does want to weigh 100. I guess there are two questions I have for you: one, of course, is whether this is good enough. I sense some exaggeration on the issue of periods; she knows this is a key measure we are waiting for. The second question is what I shall tell her parents. They are very anxious to know about her, and she doesn't want them to be prying into her business. M

Dear M, Thanks for your note. I'll contact F, whom I haven't seen in a while—I was away for much of May and early June. F is obviously still restricting quite a bit and still very much in the grip of her eating disorder. My estimate is that 100 pounds is too little for her to be healthy, but it's better than where she is now. I'd estimate a healthy weight (menstruating and ovulating) for her to be closer to 115 pounds—she's 5'4". She's very reluctant to take medication (refuses) and hasn't been willing/able to drive down here for regular meetings (in part because I think she knows what she's likely to hear from and be asked by me). I think you should clearly reinforce the negative health consequences for her re bones, reproductive function, cardiac function, etc.; be encouraging; and have her come in frequently for weighings and, if she's purging, K+ values or rhythm strips. Re speaking with her family, she's now 23 years old and therefore legally has the right to privacy—if the family asks you might just say, "F doesn't want me to discuss this with you—you should ask her directly and/or get her permission for me to speak with you." That in itself should alert them to the fact that her progress has come to a screeching halt. I hope this helps—please keep me informed and let me know if I can assist in any way. JY

E-Mail to Intervene in a Crisis

I was asked to perform a second-opinion consultation on G, a 35-year-old professional woman living in a remote part of the state, more than 300 miles from Albuquerque. She had a long, complex psychiatric history, starting at age 16. In addition to anorexia nervosa with binge-eating/purging features and severe ongoing bulimia nervosa, she had a history of severe depressions with self-mutilation and several suicide attempts, possible bipolar disorder, and probable borderline personality disorder. She was being treated in her home community with weekly psychotherapy by a caring, competent psychologist and was being managed psychopharmacologically by a local psychiatrist. I saw her for two hours on a Tuesday and ended the consultation by telling her what I thought her problems were, mentioning several elements that might benefit her treatment program, and promising to contact her psychologist and, later, her psychiatrist, who was on vacation at the time. Her psychologist and I played phone tag for a few days. Late that Friday afternoon, just before I was to leave the office, I received the following e-mail (note that use of all capital letters is sometimes the Internet equivalent of shouting):

I'M SUCH A MESS, ALMOST TOO MUCH OF A MESS FOR THERAPY. THE LINES KEEP SHIFTING AND I CAN'T KEEP UP. I CAN'T CONTAIN MYSELF. I HAVE SUCH SADNESS IN ME, CUTTING MYSELF ONLY RELEASES SOME OF WHAT IS HURTING. I'M AFRAID THAT THE ONLY WAY TO BE FREE FROM THE PAIN IS TO BLEED UNTIL I'M DONE, FINISHED. I WISH THAT I HAD BEEN ABLE TO RECEIVE THE KIND OF THERAPY I'M GETTING NOW WHEN I WAS MUCH YOUNGER, I MIGHT HAVE HAD A CHANCE. THE SHAME SEEMED ALMOST INNATE, I THINK IT WAS THE HIDDEN PART OF MY FATHER THAT I CARRIED. I THINK THAT I WAS SOMEHOW VERY SENSITIVE AND I ABSORBED WHAT WAS HAPPENING WITHOUT REALLY KNOWING JUST WHAT IT WAS. IT SEEMED THAT IT CAME FROM INSIDE OF ME, I DIDN'T HAVE ENOUGH PERSPECTIVE TO EXPERIENCE IT ANY OTHER WAY. THAT "SEED" GREW OVER THE YEARS AND CONFIRMED ITS EXISTANCE OVER AND OVER AGAIN THROUGH VARIOUS EXPERIENCES—THE LAST INCIDENT BEING THE FINAL NAIL IN MY COFFIN. I JUST KNOW THAT I'VE EXPERIENCED THIS DEPRESSION FOR MOST OF MY LIFE. I'M NOT SO SURE I'LL MAKE IT THROUGH THIS, IT HAS GONE ON FOR SO LONG AND I AM TIRED. G

In this case, I didn't want to waste any time with e-mail. I immediately tried phoning G, who wasn't at home. I tried phoning her psychologist, but she wasn't available, either. Knowing that her psychiatrist was on vacation, I phoned her office to try to get in touch with the person covering and was directed to a mental health center. I told the nurse on duty there about the patient, and she agreed to try to get in touch with the psychologist and with the patient, and to arrange for local assessment and intervention. Finally, after making these calls, I responded to the patient's e-mail as follows:

Hi, G. Please hold on, and please call your psychologist and try to reach your psychiatrist's back-up. If you can't reach them and you're really feeling very suicidal, please get yourself to a local hospital for some care. I tried reaching you by phone but got no answer. I also got answering machines at your psychologist's and your psychiatrist's offices. I called your psychiatrist's back-up emergency number and reached a nurse at the mental health center who will try to contact your psychologist and have her get in touch with you ASAP. Please let me know how you do with this. Best wishes and good luck! JY

I was not able to reach her psychologist that night. The next morning, I received the following e-mail from G:

> Dear Dr. Y, I just wanted you to know that I managed to get through my crisis, I've talked to my psychologist several times over the last 24 hours and I think I'm a little more clear now. My psychiatrist is out of town for two weeks. I've been off my Depakote for over two weeks now. I'm taking Klonopin twice a day and Prozac once in the morning. I decided to start taking an extra Prozac every other day. I don't know how important it is that I be on an additional medication like the one you suggested during our visit. I'm assuming it's ok to wait until my psychiatrist has returned?? Thank you for getting me help yesterday. I hate it when I become so disjointed and needy. I'm sad to have that part of me back ... or maybe she's been there all along, just hiding in the shadows. It's so hard to work at getting well when I can't figure out what's real and what isn't. Anyway, I just wanted to let you know that I'm steady now and that I will continue to work with my psychologist to find my way out of this. Thanks again. G

> *Hi, G. Thanks so much for letting me know how you are. I really appreciate it, and I'm glad that you've managed to get through the crisis. My sense is that your psychologist is working well with you. Re medication, I don't think anything urgent needs to happen, but if you're still feeling very shaky there are certain medications you're not taking now that may help. I should talk with your psychiatrist about options when she gets back. In the meantime, I'll also try to speak with your psychologist. Best wishes, and good luck! JY*

I spoke with her psychologist at length the following Monday.

Discussion

E-mail appears to have been helpful to at least some extent in each of these cases, and in none has the patient or I experienced any negative effects from including e-mail in the treatment (other than relatively minor reactions, such as B's resentment at having to check in). In every instance, e-mail was only one component of a more elaborate treatment plan. Of the patients with whom I've used e-mail, several have been in concurrent ongoing individual psychotherapy with a therapist, have had intermittent visits with a dietician, and/or have been taking psychotropic medications. In several cases, family members have also been involved. Given this assortment of interventions, it's difficult to tease out the specific contributions of e-mail to the overall effectiveness of treatment. However, the adjunctive use of e-mail in the therapeutic process raises several general issues for consideration.

Potential Benefits of Adjunctive E-Mail

Patients' comments suggest several facilitory factors. E-mail concretely increases the frequency and amount of contact between patients and clinicians. Giving patients even brief feedback several times a week between sessions lets them know that their clinicians are present, listening, and thinking about them. From this perspective, clinicians need to inform their patients about their e-mail habits, specifically how often they read e-mail and how often they are likely to respond. Such information prepares patients for what they might expect with regard to the timing of responses from their clinicians. The frequency, length, and responsiveness of e-mail contact all increase patients' sense of being in touch with and touched by their clinicians. The amount of time that patients devote to composing e-mails to their clinicians, although variable, is sometimes considerable. It takes a reasonable amount of time to think about what to write and to physically type messages. Some are faster typists than others, and some write more fluidly (and expressively) than others. Ordinarily, much less time is required for clinicians to read and respond to their patients' messages.

E-mail enables patients to write and send messages whenever inspiration strikes. Rather than being forced to engage with clinicians according to fixed schedules, patients can write their e-mail messages when they're most inclined to do so. E-mail offers on-demand feeding. Having their messages read later is less important than being able to initiate contact at any time. It is important to feel heard, and having an imagined e-mail "ear" available all the time adds to the sense of being held and contained. Patients may even come to feel that they have virtually constant access to their clinicians. The emotional value of these communications is often increased because patients initiate them when they feel most needy and interested, when they most desire to be in contact with their clinicians, and when they are most cathected to the process. Because they are explicitly invited to correspond via e-mail and know that their messages will be read only when convenient, they don't have to worry about interrupting their clinicians or intruding on their clinicians' private time. Many patients are highly loath to impose themselves on their clinicians, especially if they fear that their clinicians might respond by feeling put upon or upset. Thus, access without guilt is a clear benefit of the asynchronous nature of e-mail (Negroponte, 1996).

E-mail reduces the emotional burden on patients by making it easier for them to say what's on their minds. Patients have greater control over e-mail and thus worry less about inadvertently giving away emotional signals. Computers benignly and approvingly accept whatever patients care to reveal—all their confessions, admonitions, and quirky ideas—and do so without interrupting them. Social psychologists and sociologists who have studied computer-based communications have found that individuals often feel much freer writing to a computer than talking to a person (Negroponte, 1996; Turkel, 1984, 1995).* Patients may use e-mail to expand on, reconstruct, repair, or annotate what they say in person, to try to ensure that they communicate what they want to. Patients are more likely to open up if they don't have to be on the alert for and react to their clinicians' moment-to-moment comments or body language. As is evident in several of the messages in this chapter, some patients may interact less formally via e-mail than in person. I've never been called Dr. Yagermeister or Dr. Dude to my face; these terms clearly became affectionate (and endearing) appellations via e-mail. (In my view, when clinicians respond via e-mail, it's important to respect and foster their patients' less formal styles of communication.) We know that individuals can establish meaningful and even powerful relationships online. Furthermore, when a clinician explicitly invites a patient to e-mail, that authorization to initiate contact enhances the patient's autonomy in the therapeutic relationship, decreasing the power differential between them.

One of the most potent aspects of using quasi-daily e-mail in treating patients with anorexia nervosa is that this reporting arrangement forces patients to be constantly aware of their behaviors and of being in therapy. Some patients admit that they easily become inattentive to therapeutic expectations between office visits. Having to report in demands that they honestly think about and confront their own behaviors on a more frequent basis. C found this aspect of frequent e-mail contact to be particularly vexing but effective. Also, when patients provide their clinicians with certain details via e-mail, for example, calorie counts or behavior or symptom logs, office time that would be devoted to reviewing this information is freed for discussion of more meaningful issues.

Given the various demographic and clinical characteristics of anorexia nervosa, adjunctive e-mail therapy may, theoretically, be particularly well suited for women with this disorder. First, many patients are adolescents and young adults, and arguably the majority now has knowledge about and access to computers; they belong to the demographic groups most likely to use e-mail. Second, talking to a computer may be especially beneficial and relatively easier for patients with anorexia nervosa, whose obedient, compliant, self-proclaimedly honest, diligent, harm-avoidant, shy, timid personalities are likely to adhere to an e-mail regimen. E-mail may diminish some of the social awkwardness and transferential difficulties such patients experience in person, where—based

---

*It's possible that being online evokes other aspects of our "protean" selves (Lifton, 1993) that are usually expressed in face-to-face contact. Through this, the therapist may get an expanded view of the patient's being.

on what they perceive to be their clinicians' attitudes and reactions of the moment—their exquisite interpersonal sensitivities may cause them to inhibit, restrain, or alter their expression of spontaneous ideas and emotions. Patients with anorexia nervosa tend to be shy and often have some degree of social phobia, problems that may lend themselves to e-mail-mediated interventions (King & Poulos, 1998). Some patients with anorexia nervosa have trouble looking a clinician in the eye, but not in the computer. Their intuitive sense that adding e-mail contact to treatment is a good thing manifests in the flash of interest, excitement, and general eagerness to participate that occurs in most instances when I suggest such contact. Patients experience the invitation to e-mail as a sign that their clinicians are interested in how they are doing outside of scheduled office sessions, or recognize the value of more contact than weekly office sessions ordinarily permit. My perception is that many patients also sense that this mode of communication will be comfortable and work for them. The impact of these relationships on patients' transference reactions to their clinicians is worthy of further study. In my experience, adjunctive e-mail has almost always increased positive transference.

Responding Appropriately to E-Mail From Patients

In general, my responses provide brief comments on what patients have written about, acknowledge their struggles with these tough disorders, and include words of encouragement. When patients are demoralized, I provide a positive perspective that supports their self-esteem and pride, and on very special occasions I offer a "virtual hug"—which in my opinion does not constitute a boundary violation. On those infrequent occasions, as with G, when a patient writes about something particularly distressing or pressing and I feel that a brief e-mail response will not suffice, I phone the patient and either spend a few minutes on the phone to clarify the issue or schedule an additional office visit.

Potential Negative Consequences of Adjunctive E-Mail

Although infrequent in my experience, potential negative effects of e-mail therapy may include:

> Unwanted disclosures resulting from lack of privacy when receiving e-mail messages. This may be a particular risk if the patient shares a computer or an e-mail address with other family members, as did A, and the clinician either includes the patient's message in his or her reply or fails to reply in a nonspecific, discreet manner.

Failure by the clinician to recognize urgent, troubled communications. E-mail may not suffice for assessment or reassurance, and phone and/or face-to-face contact may be merited.

Failure by the clinician to respond in a timely or adequate fashion. Even when there isn't a crisis, this can leave the patient feeling neglected.

Excessive or otherwise inappropriate messages from the patient. Such issues would always be subject to discussion in person, as would other transference-related communications.

In addition, resistance to using e-mail is, in my experience, an early and strong predictor of generalized resistance to treatment and as such adds to the overall clinical information available to the provider. This early warning signal should generate appropriate discussion with the patient and often indicates the need for additional motivational enhancement.

Other Professional Issues

Using e-mail in the context of therapy raises legal and ethical issues concerning informed consent, confidentiality, and related matters (Rothchild, 1997; Shapiro & Schulman, 1996; Spielberg, 1998). Patients need to be reminded that e-mail is not necessarily a secure mode of communication. For reasons illustrated by the clinical examples I have provided, patients should always be encouraged to use private rather than shared e-mail addresses and be advised not to write anything they wouldn't want other people to see. Negroponte (1996) felicitously referred to this as practicing "safe text." Prompted by the Health Insurance Portability and Accountability Act regulations regarding patient confidentiality, I have now established a Web site for my practice using Medem (www.medem.com), a company supported by numerous medical societies including the American Psychiatric Association (APA) and the American Medical Association (AMA). Members of the American Psychiatric Association can create, without charge, Web sites that include encrypted electronic communication. The procedures for setting up the system are relatively simple. Some authorities strongly suggest that patients sign separate informed consent forms if e-mail is to be routinely employed (Spielberg, 1998). Patients should also know that messages sent via e-mail may be saved in some aspect of their medical records.

Clearly, e-therapy is an emerging business, and professionals will want to charge for their time. In my experience, using e-mail as an adjunct for treating anorexia nervosa is still untested, and because I have not had to spend an inordinate amount of time reading or responding to e-mail messages, I have not yet billed for e-mail services. However, the time a therapist spends on e-mail with a patient may turn out, in the aggregate, to be considerable relative to the time spent with the patient in the office. The amount of time expended may ultimately justify "bundling" charges for e-mail services together with office visits to determine an overall fee for outpatient care.

Future Applications of E-Mail in Treating Patients With Eating Disorders

The use of e-mail in psychotherapy is still in its infancy (literature searches on Medline and PsycInfo still elicit very few articles addressing these issues). The promising results of this small case series suggest a number of future directions.

Several recent studies of outpatient treatment for anorexia nervosa have revealed relatively disappointing outcomes (Bergh, Eriksson, Lindberg, & Sodersten, 1996), and studies employing cognitive-behavioral therapy for anorexia nervosa have shown high rates of dropouts (K. A. Halmi, J. E. Mitchell, W. S. Agras, personal communications, October, 2001). It is possible that adding e-mail as an adjunct to psychotherapy in person may increase adherence and effectiveness for the reasons provided earlier. Systematic research is needed to determine whether adjunctive e-mail treatment might benefit not only those receiving cognitive-behavioral therapy for anorexia nervosa (in which e-mail may take care of some diary-keeping business), but other kinds of outpatient treatment as well, including interpersonal psychotherapy and family psychotherapies. Controlled trials may help elucidate the potential utility of adjunctive e-mail therapy in such treatments.

Computers have recently been used in college-based preventive interventions to engage and to help individuals with early or subclinical eating disorders (Winzelberg et al., 1998). Studies have also shown that a sizeable minority of patients with bulimia nervosa or binge-eating disorder may benefit from using guided self-help, based on professionally written manuals, that sufferers may use with or without additional professional support (Hartley, 1995; Rathner, Bonsch, Maurer, Walter, & Sollner, 1993). E-mail-based review and support programs may be fruitfully linked to these manuals. Early pilot studies have also indicated that some patients with clinical bulimia nervosa, binge-eating disorder, and "eating disorders, not otherwise specified" may benefit from e-mail therapy based on cognitive-behavioral principles (Robertson, as reported in Sherman, 2000). Trials to study the potentially increased impact of manuals plus e-mail should be investigated.

A number of e-mail-based groups for people with eating disorders already exist (Holmes, 1998). To my knowledge, no systematic assessment has been conducted of the impact that these programs have on those who participate. Preliminary studies of psychiatric consumers with other diagnoses—including schizophrenia, bipolar illness, and major depression—have shown that e-mail support groups may be extremely educational, motivational, and helpful (Pederson, Warner, & Yager, 1999).

To summarize, I have started to routinely offer the use of e-mail as an adjunct to the outpatient treatment of patients with anorexia nervosa. Preliminary evaluation suggests a high degree of patient acceptability and adherence. Patients who take advantage of this modality report benefits due to the increased contact with me, the ad-lib availability of the computer as confessor, and their daily confrontation of their own integrity and eating-related behaviors. Relatively little clinician time is required to read and respond to e-mails, and the potential clinical benefits appear to justify this allocation of professional resources. There are evident limits to e-mail therapy. Those patients who are resistant to treatment in general will also be resistant to using e-mail because the requirement of frequent reporting makes their difficulties in engaging all the move obvious to them and to their clinicians. Controlled trials to better evaluate the potential contributions of e-mail to different populations receiving varied modalities of psychotherapies and other outpatient treatments are needed and would be most welcome.

References

Bergh, C., Eriksson, M., Lindberg, G., & Sodersten, P. (1996). Selective serotonin reuptake inhibitors in anorexia. *Lancet, 348*(9039), 1459–1460.

Dunham, P. J., Hurshman, A., Litwin, E., Gusella, J., Ellsworth, C., & Dodd, P. W. D. (1998). Computer-mediated social support: Single young mothers as a model system. *American Journal of Community Psychology, 26*, 281–306.

Hartley, P. (1995). Changing body image through guided self-help: A pilot study. *Eating Disorders: The Journal of Treatment & Prevention, 3*(2), 165–174.

Holmes, L. G. (1998). Delivering mental health services on-line: Current issues. *Cyberpsychology & Behavior, 1*(1), 19–24.

Kiesler, S., Siegel, J., & McGuire, T. (1984). Social psychological aspects of computer-mediated communication. *American Psychologist, 39*, 1123–1134.

King, S. A., & Poulos, S. T. (1998). Using the internet to treat generalized social phobia and avoidant personality disorder. *CyberPsychology & Behavior, 1*, 29–36.

Lifton, R. J. (1993). *The protean self: Human resilience in an age of fragmentation.* New York: Basic Books.

Murphy, L. J., & Mitchell, D. L. (1998). When writing helps to heal: E-mail as therapy. *British Journal of Guidance & Counselling, 26*(1), 21–32.

Negroponte, N. (1996). *Being digital.* New York: Vintage/Random House.

Pederson, C., Warner, T., & Yager, J. (1999). Unpublished data.

Rathner, G., Bonsch, C., Maurer, G., Walter, M. H., & Sollner, W. (1993). The impact of a "guided self-help group" on bulimic women: A prospective 15 month study of attenders and non-attenders. *Journal of Psychosomatic Research, 37*(4), 389–396.

Rothchild, E. (1997). E-mail therapy. *American Journal of Psychiatry, 154,* 1476–1477.

Shapiro, D. E., & Schulman C. E. (1996). Ethical and legal issues in e-mail therapy. *Ethics and Behavior, 6,* 107–124.

Sherman, C. (2000, July). Eating disorder patients receptive to e-mail therapy. *Clinical Psychiatry News, 28*(7), 23.

Spielberg, A. R. (1998). On call and online: Sociohistorical, legal, and ethical implications of e-mail for the patient–physician relationship. *JAMA, 280,* 1353–1359.

Stroh, M. (1999, June 5). Doctors make modern house calls over the Internet. *The Albuquerque Journal,* pp. C1, C2.

Turkel, S. (1984). *The second self: Computers and the human spirit.* New York: Simon & Shuster.

Turkel, S. (1995). *Life on the screen: Identity in the age of the Internet.* New York: Simon & Shuster.

Wilson, G., & Lester, D. (1998). Suicide prevention by e-mail. *Crisis Intervention & Time-Limited Treatment, 4,* 81–87.

Winzelberg, A. J., Taylor, C. B., Sharpe, T., Eldredge, K. L., Dev, P., & Constantinou, P. S. (1998). Evaluation of a computer-mediated eating disorder intervention program. *International Journal of Eating Disorders, 24,* 339–349.

4

A Model Community Telepsychiatry Program in Rural Arizona

*Sara F. Gibson, Susan Morley,
and Catherine P. Romeo-Wolff*

INTEREST IN THE USE of videoconferencing to provide medical services has surged throughout the United States and the world in recent years. Because psychiatry utilizes primarily verbal modalities as diagnostic and therapeutic tools, and does not require hands-on procedures, it has been at the forefront of this movement. Often referred to as "telemedicine" or "telepsychiatry," videoconferencing has been touted as a solution to the problems of providing psychiatric access to medically underserved, primarily rural areas in which the cost of transporting either clients or psychiatrists is prohibitive.

In 1996, Northern Arizona Regional Behavioral Health Authority established a videoconferencing system to increase the availability of behavioral health services throughout northern Arizona. Special emphasis was placed on the provision of services to low-income, indigent, or uninsured persons in medically underserved (primarily rural and sparsely populated) areas. Since December 1996, Little Colorado Behavioral Health Centers in Apache County has provided all outpatient psychiatric care (all physician–patient contact) solely via this telemedicine system. Other northern Arizona clinics have provided a combination of on-site (face-to-face) psychiatry and telepsychiatry.

Description of the Program

NARBHA Overview

Northern Arizona Regional Behavioral Health Authority (NARBHA) was founded in 1967 as a private, nonprofit corporation. It originally provided administrative support for seven local community mental health centers in the five northern Arizona counties. As Arizona's behavioral health system began receiving Medicaid funding in the early 1990s, the Arizona Department of Health Services designated NARBHA as the managed care organization responsible for the northern region of the state.

Since its inception, NARBHA has placed a high priority on developing community-based behavioral health services. To make behavioral health services readily accessible in communities throughout this rural region, NARBHA contracts with behavioral health service providers (referred to as Service Area Agencies) located in 22 communities in northern Arizona (see Figure 4.1). In outpatient, residential, and inpatient settings, these agencies provide comprehensive behavioral health care to adults, children, families, alcohol- and drug-use clients, and the seriously mentally ill.

Drivers for the Establishment of a Telemedicine System

With a vast (62,000 square miles), rural, and sparsely populated (475,000 people) region, NARBHA faced numerous difficulties in delivering behavioral health services:

- Specialized staff (psychiatrists and other behavioral health professionals) were not available in all communities.
- Agencies with multiple locations had staff traveling on a regular basis anywhere from 30 minutes to $2\frac{1}{2}$ hours between sites in order to provide evaluation/diagnosis, case management, and direct treatment services.
- Training and continuing education opportunities were limited.
- Consultation with other psychiatrists and participation in peer review activities for psychiatrists were not possible.
- Staff members felt professionally isolated, adding to high turnover and recruitment difficulties.
- The time spent traveling greatly reduced the time spent delivering direct client services.

In the late 1980s, NARBHA heard that local community colleges and Northern Arizona University were developing a system to provide education over a

FIGURE 4.1
NARBHA SITES.

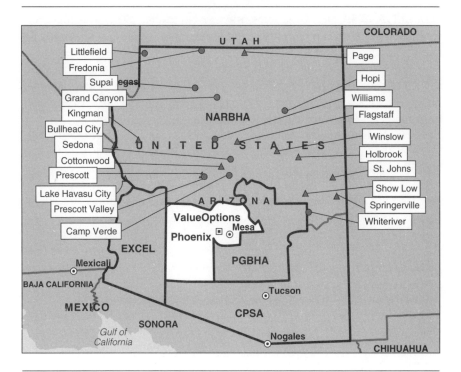

microwave-based videoconferencing system. At the time it seemed too futuristic, but NARBHA knew that videoconferencing technology could also help in the delivery of behavioral health services. Although these early discussions did not result in NARBHA utilizing those fledgling systems, NARBHA began following the development of the technology and saw the telemedicine industry blossom. By 1994, NARBHA's interest had grown to the point of having several vendors demonstrate their equipment. However, at that point the prevailing judgment was that the picture transmission, still at 15 frames per second, was insufficient for delivering quality psychiatric services.

In the spring of 1995, Arizona State House Bill 2275 allocated the annual amount of $250,000 of tobacco tax revenues to establish a telemedicine pilot program to facilitate the provision of medical services to low-income, indigent, or uninsured persons living in medically underserved areas of Arizona.

NARBHA proposed a system to enhance the delivery of behavioral health services in Northern Arizona and, in January 1996, received their first allocation of $250,000 from the Arizona Department of Health Services. The system, dubbed NARBHA Net, began operation in November 1996, utilizing dedicated T1 lines between clinic sites and connecting to a hub in Flagstaff. By adding other state and local funding, NARBHA Net began with six video-conference sites. The end of 1997 brought six more sites, and early 1998 the latest two. In mid-1998, NARBHA assisted another one of the Regional Behavioral Health Authorities, Community Partnership of Southern Arizona, in bringing up their own eight-site network and linked the two networks at the Arizona Department of Health Services Division of Behavioral Health Services, in Phoenix, where yet another site was also added. In the fall of 1998, NARBHA established a permanent network connection to the University of Arizona Telemedicine Program for the purpose of receiving weekly psychiatric grand rounds, which enabled clinical staff at the Regional Behavioral Health Authorities to earn continuing medical education credits. This link also increased the availability of specialty consultation from the University. At about that same time, a third Regional Behavioral Health Authority, Pinal Gila Behavioral Health Association (PGBHA), linked one site in Apache Junction to the "mini-hub" located at Behavioral Health Services in Phoenix, becoming part of the growing statewide network of networks (see Table 4.1).

NARBHA Net Description

TECHNICAL DETAILS
In selecting video equipment, a team of NARBHA staff—including Teresa Bertsch, MD, Medical Director, and Susan Morley, MSW, CISW, Director of Telemedicine Programs—tested several telemedicine systems to evaluate different bandwidths, speeds, and features. NARBHA was committed to ensuring clinical quality and, as part of the equipment selection process, Dr. Bertsch tested the equipment's ability to allow the performance of the Abnormal Involuntary Movement Scale (AIMS), a visual, scored, standardized examination that psychiatrists routinely perform to look for side effects (especially tardive dyskinesia) of antipsychotics. Dr. Bertsch performed mock AIMS tests on people at distant sites—zooming in on their mouths to look for lip pursing, having them stick their tongues and stretch their hands out to look for tremors, and zooming out to watch their gaits. Based on this evaluation of the equipment, Dr. Bertsch proposed a very high transmission rate of 512 kilobits per second (8 channels; the industry standard at that time was 384 kbps, 6 channels), which provided 30 frames per second with excellent picture quality. Although some may argue that 512 kbps was more bandwidth than necessary, each

TABLE 4.1
NARBHA Net Sites

YEAR OF ADDITION	LOCATION OF SITE
1996	Flagstaff (hub) Show Low St. Johns Page Prescott Arizona State Hospital, Phoenix
1997	Flagstaff (second site) Springerville Holbrook Kingman Lake Havasu City Winslow
1998	Bullhead City Cottonwood Behavioral Health Services, Phoenix (mini-hub) University of Arizona, Tucson Community Partnership of Southern Arizona, Tucson (regional network)
1999	Pinal Gila Behavioral Health Association, Apache Junction

additional channel of video provided smoother flow of motion and less image degradation.

UTILIZATION

The telemedicine system is in near-constant use at multiple sites during the workweek (see Table 4.2). During its first full year of operation (1997), over 90% of videoconferences were for clinical use. In 1998, the number of clinical

TABLE 4.2
Types of NARBHA Net Use

YEAR	NUMBER OF VIDEOCONFERENCES (% OF TOTAL VIDEOCONFERENCES)		
	CLINICAL	ADMINISTRATIVE	EDUCATIONAL
1997	841 (91.5%)	51 (5.5%)	27 (3.0%)
1998	1647 (91.0%)	133 (7.3%)	31 (1.7%)
1999	1992 (87.3%)	229 (10.0%)	60 (2.6%)

sessions doubled. In 1999, the increase in clinical use was not as dramatic, but still significant (almost 18%). There is not a meeting or training session that we don't attempt to conduct using videoconferencing. Telemedicine is the way we conduct our particular business in northern Arizona.

Clinical Uses

LITTLE COLORADO BEHAVIORAL HEALTH CENTERS, APACHE COUNTY

Apache County is a large, sparsely populated, rural county in northeastern Arizona, bordering New Mexico. Of the 11,216 square miles in the county, the Navajo Indian Reservation comprises 65%. The nearest metropolitan area is Flagstaff (population 50,000, and a 2- or 3-hour drive away). Little Colorado Behavioral Health Centers, the local Service Area Agency, is responsible for providing behavioral health services to approximately 15,000 off-reservation residents. Because of its remote, rural location, its pair of clinics (St. Johns and Springerville) have traditionally struggled to recruit psychiatrists to work there part time. In 1996, the local psychiatrist retired, again putting the clinic in a recruitment crisis. Only 15 to 20 hours a week of psychiatrist time were needed, and because efforts to recruit a psychiatrist to move to the county had failed, the options seemed limited to flying a psychiatrist in from Phoenix once a month or transporting clients to a neighboring county to see a psychiatrist. Sara Gibson, MD, who was working at NARBHA in an administrative role, agreed to provide psychiatric services for the Apache County clinics over the newly established NARBHA Net. A seamless transition between psychiatrists occurred, and continuous medical service was maintained.

Since December 1996, Dr. Gibson has provided all psychiatric evaluations and medication followups, attended all inpatient and outpatient staffings, and performed all medical director duties from the NARBHA Net hub in Flagstaff. Clients are seen in Springerville, 180 miles away, on Wednesdays. The hookup with St. Johns, which is 150 miles from Flagstaff, is on Thursdays.

Upon presentation to the clinic, a client sees an intake worker and is assigned to a therapist or case manager on site. If referred for psychiatric evaluation or medication management, the client is oriented to the telemedicine system both in writing and verbally, and signs a videoconference consent form (see the appendices to this chapter). Twenty-five to thirty percent of clients seen in Apache County for counseling are referred for psychiatric care. The therapist or case manager accompanies the client to all telemedicine sessions (with rare exceptions) and participates in the evaluation and management as a member of the treatment team. Families are welcomed into sessions, along

TABLE 4.3
1999 NARBHA Net Client Demographics

Total # of clinical videoconferences	1992
Number of clients	1268
Gender	M = 597 (47%) F = 671 (53%)
Ethnicity	White = 869 (68.5%) Black = 32 (2.5%) Hispanic = 201 (15.9%) Native American = 67 (5.3%) Other = 43 (3.4%) Unaccounted for = 56 (4.4%)*
Subpopulation	Serious mental illness = 507 (40.0%) Mental health = 228 (18.0%) Alcohol abuse = 56 (4.4%) Drug abuse = 58 (4.6%) Children = 407 (32.1%) Other = 12 (0.9%)

*Data was not reported on ethnicity for these clients.

with other involved parties (probation officers, school staff, caseworkers from other agencies, etc.).

All Apache County clients requiring outpatient psychiatric services are seen over NARBHA Net, whether for the initial psychiatric evaluation, or subsequent medication followups, or case management staffings. Half of the clients meet Arizona's diagnostic criteria for "serious mental illness." One quarter are children, and another quarter are adults with general mental health or substance abuse disorders (see Table 4.3).

Adult clients requiring inpatient care are generally sent 60 miles away to an acute care inpatient facility in Show Low. Because Show Low is also on NARBHA Net, weekly three-way videoconference staffings occur involving the psychiatrist in Flagstaff, the inpatient team and the client in Show Low, and the case manager or therapist and sometimes family members in Apache County. The ability to involve all parties has greatly facilitated discharge planning.

Medical recordkeeping is difficult and has required an increase in services from support staff. The original, full chart resides in Apache County. In Flagstaff, the psychiatrist keeps a second chart that contains all information deemed immediately necessary to provide care, including copies of current medical and psychiatric notes, laboratory results, and old records. After seeing a client, a copy of the psychiatrist's note is made for the Flagstaff record, and the original is faxed or mailed to Apache County to be inserted into the full chart. Digital health records are being explored and, if implemented, will alleviate many of these recordkeeping difficulties. Laboratory results are faxed or mailed from Apache County to Flagstaff; prescriptions are called, faxed, or mailed from Flagstaff to Apache County. For a Schedule II medication, which requires the original prescription, an inevitable delay occurs while it is mailed. Clients are alerted to this potential delay and are asked to notify staff in advance of running out of medications. Collaboration with local pharmacists has been essential to streamlining this system. Medication samples cannot be kept at the Apache County sites because medical personnel are not physically present, so coupons are used or, rarely, medication samples are mailed.

Apache County primary care physicians and other health care providers have been integral to the success of the telemedicine system. Because no medical personnel work at the Apache County sites, any client who requires assessment in person must be referred to their primary care provider. Blood pressure, pulse, and weight are monitored in Apache County by therapists, but questionable results are evaluated by local medical personnel. Frequent phone calls and collaboration are essential, and local primary care providers have been pleased to facilitate this process. They, in turn, appreciate the availability of psychiatric expertise in the county.

Other clinical applications have evolved utilizing the telemedicine system. Psychiatrists throughout the system cover for vacationing colleagues and fill in when staff vacancies occur. Subspecialist consultations are obtained from the University of Arizona in Tucson, and from a neuropsychiatrist at Arizona State Hospital in Phoenix. Clients simply go to their local Service Area Agency and are evaluated by the subspecialist in Phoenix or Tucson, at a great time and cost savings. The referring psychiatrist can also attend from Flagstaff over NARBHA Net to enhance communication and continuity of care.

Some Service Area Agencies do employ local psychiatrists. Board-certified child and adolescent psychiatrists are especially difficult to recruit, so most children in northern Arizona are seen by general psychiatrists. It has been invaluable to have the telemedicine system available to use for consultations with child psychiatrists employed at other Service Area Agencies on more difficult child and adolescent cases. The child, his or her family, and the local treating psychiatrist can remain in their home community and simply hook up with the specialist over NARBHA Net for the consultation. A complete evaluation takes place, and recommendations are passed back to the local treating psychiatrist for ongoing care. Followup consultations are easily arranged. The patient and parents are pleased to have access to the subspecialist, and the local psychiatrist is pleased to have the consultation both from clinical and medical-legal perspectives.

ARIZONA STATE HOSPITAL

Arizona has one state psychiatric hospital, located in Phoenix. A client from northern Arizona who is admitted there is managed by the Service Area Agency in his or her home community. This requires the case manager and state hospital liaison from the local Service Area Agency to meet with the Arizona State Hospital clinical team—consisting of a social worker, a vocation rehabilitation coordinator, a nursing coordinator, and an attending psychiatrist—and the client on a monthly basis. The Service Area Agency psychiatrist, who will be the outpatient treating psychiatrist, may also attend. These meetings improve coordination of care and are utilized to discuss the admission, the medical necessity of continued inpatient treatment, and discharge planning. The client, his or her family, and the local psychiatrist may also meet with the treatment team of the state hospital, before the admission and after discharge, to facilitate the transitions. The NARBHA Net connection at the state hospital is also utilized for informal hearings when discharge planning problems arise, to enable participation from client advocates and other staff from various northern Arizona locations.

Because these staffings are an important part of the admission and discharge processes, NARBHA chose the state hospital as one of its first six videoconference sites, purchasing the room equipment for that facility. With as many as 15 case staffings per month, staff travel to Phoenix was inefficient; it required a whole day, with travel time, to participate in a 30- to 45-minute case conference. Although there were early difficulties in transporting clients from the psychiatric units on the grounds of the hospital to the building in which the videoconferencing equipment was housed, these issues have been successfully resolved. The state hospital is currently designing a new hospital and is planning for videoconference rooms in various locations in the new facility.

OTHER CLINICAL USES

Videoconferencing is also used regularly when a client is placed in a residential treatment facility out of his or her area. Because there are no residential treatment facilities for children in northern Arizona, a child or adolescent requiring residential treatment is placed a long distance away, usually in Phoenix. The staffings involve the treatment team and the child at the residential facility; the Service Area Agency, school staff, and the family in the home community; and juvenile corrections and child welfare personnel who may be located in communities other than the client's primary community. Increased participation by collateral agencies has occurred now that time and distance factors have largely been eliminated. Videoconferencing allows all team members and many family members to participate. Thanks to NARBHA Net, families can "visit" their children without driving, round trip, for six to eight hours (and often missing work or having to find child care for other children in the home).

Videoconferencing has been used to provide e-therapy when it is determined to be clinically advantageous (e.g., a client developed a strong therapeutic relationship with a therapist, moved to a new location, and was considered high risk). However, because most Service Area Agencies have adequate therapist and case management staffing, e-therapy usage has been limited.

Training and Educational Uses

Providing training throughout the NARBHA region has been an ongoing challenge. Obtaining continuing medical education credits used to require out-of-town travel for NARBHA psychiatrists and other clinical staff. Because of the time, distance, and expense—as well as the need to maintain service provision and crisis coverage while staff were away from their work site—only a limited number of staff had been able to participate in off-site educational activities. In order to minimize the impact of travel time, NARBHA only provided training or clinical education to its Service Area Agency staff when there was enough content for a 6- to 8-hour program.

Arizona State Hospital was selected as an initial NARBHA Net site because of both the clinical cost savings and the frequent training and education that was provided there and could be offered to staff in northern Arizona. The added training and educational opportunities were an immediate benefit to staff.

In 1998, NARBHA Net connected to the University of Arizona Telemedicine Program. Sites in the two networks seamlessly link to each other for clinical consultation and administrative meetings. Weekly psychiatric grand rounds that provide continuing education for psychiatrists and other clinical staff throughout the region have been well received by NARBHA staff. One clinical psychiatrist said, "Not only do we listen to and see the speaker presentations, we are also able to participate in discussions and receive CME and other professional credits on a weekly basis, free, and in the comfort of our local clinic telemedicine site."

Through videoconferences, NARBHA itself has been able to provide additional training and educational activities for clinical and administrative staff at its Service Area Agencies. With travel time no longer an issue, frequent 1- to

3-hour training and educational events have become the norm. An 8-week family therapy training session, provided for child and family therapists throughout the region, allowed a group of staff to meet weekly and was highly successful. In addition, Service Area Agencies with multiple sites throughout the county regularly videoconference for internal staff training and education. NARBHA and the other rural Regional Behavioral Health Authorities formed the Greater Arizona Training Alliance, whose goal is to offer high-quality training and educational opportunities with nationally recognized speakers to rural sites through videoconferences. Its first systemwide training, in January 2000, linked 24 sites and hundreds of participants throughout the entire state for $1\frac{1}{2}$ days of training by an expert in schizophrenia. One day of the training was geared specifically to consumers, family members, and advocates, and the use of videoconferencing made the training accessible to all.

Administrative Uses

Meetings, technical assistance, and agency oversight activities that previously required staff travel now are available regularly through videoconferences. NARBHA's board of directors, which is comprised of individuals living throughout northern Arizona, meets monthly. These evening meetings used to require board members to travel long distances at night, sometimes in snowy weather. Members who live 2 to 3 hours away now regularly attend over NARBHA Net, which has increased board participation. In addition, numerous other meetings—including those of agency directors, chief financial officers, agency psychiatrists, and the MIS users group (NARBHA's computer department)—take place over NARBHA Net. Agency site visits and monitoring (by NARBHA of its Service Area Agencies, and by the Arizona Department of Health Services of NARBHA) now also take place utilizing videoconferences, which saves considerable travel time. In 2000, during NARBHA and Service Area Agency accreditation visits by the Joint Commission on Accreditation of Healthcare Organizations, videoconferences were used by surveyors to conduct various interviews. In addition, technical assistance on clinical or administrative issues is more easily obtained through videoconferences.

Future Directions

HOME HEALTH APPLICATIONS

NARBHA is embarking on a pilot program in which portable telemedicine units are brought directly to homebound people who require psychiatric services. NARBHA is looking at this for elderly, medically fragile, or agoraphobic clients.

The unit would be brought into the home by the therapist or case manager and used for psychiatric assessment and care. These units are relatively inexpensive and require only a POTS ("plain old telephone system") line (28.8–56 kbps). Although we feel that ongoing clinical care is optimal with 512 kbps, these portable units may be a way to provide medical care to the homebound who would not have to access more traditional care.

SERVICES TO THE INCARCERATED

Arizona correctional institutions, in collaboration with the University of Arizona Telemedicine Program, have successfully implemented telemedicine to increase medical services to inmates. Through NARBHA's leadership, county jails and community mental health centers are collaborating to make mental health services more available to inmates by bringing into jails a portable or semipermanent unit that can be connected to NARBHA Net.

SECLUSION AND AFTER-HOURS COVERAGE

Rural inpatient units have struggled to comply with Centers for Medicare & Medicaid Services (formerly Health Care Financing Administration) regulations that a client placed in seclusion or restraint must be seen by a physician within an hour of the order and at frequent intervals thereafter. Inpatient facilities are small throughout the NARBHA system, and often the on-call psychiatrists don't live in the same town but instead cover the facilities by phone after hours. In order to maintain compliance with this regulation, NARBHA will be placing portable telemedicine units in seclusion rooms, and on-call psychiatrists will be able to bring a second unit home in case of such an emergency.

CENTRAL OVERSIGHT AND MANAGEMENT

Under the leadership of Catherine Romeo-Wolff, NARBHA's Telemedicine Program Manager, administrative and scheduling centralization of four Regional Behavioral Health Authority telemedicine networks (those of NARBHA, Pinal Gila Behavioral Health Association, Community Partnership of Southern Arizona, and Excel Group) was initiated in 2001. This project, whose goal is to streamline processes both for users of the systems and administrative staff, economizes by using existing hub equipment and sharing new hub equipment (e.g., multipoint conferencing units).

RESEARCH

NARBHA is collaborating with the University of Arizona Telemedicine Program to research the efficacy of telemedicine in psychiatry. One study, which is just beginning, will assess the reliability of the Abnormal Involuntary Movement Scale when administered using various bandwidths.

Evaluation of the Program

Accessibility

Access to services is the primary reason NARBHA developed and extensively uses its telemedicine system as a clinical tool and is the most frequently cited reason for the integration of telemedicine into medical systems in general. It is reasonable to assume that, in a perfect world, clinicians would provide services in a real human setting, without the barriers of technology between them and clients, and that most clients would also prefer to be seen in person. But such "perfect world" access to care in rural Arizona is severely compromised, especially in Apache County. Utilizing NARBHA Net, medically unstable clients can be seen weekly (as opposed to monthly), and even more frequent visits can be arranged if needed. Such clients can stay in their own community and see their own doctor more efficiently than if they had to take the day off of work and travel to another city. Hence, their likelihood of compliance with their treatment plans is greatly enhanced.

Physician continuity is often very difficult to achieve in rural areas, which further reduces the quality of care. Northern Arizona, as a medically underserved area, is sometimes able to use National Health Service Corps loan repayment or scholarship programs to recruit psychiatrists. However, after the contract period has ended, the problem of retaining the psychiatrist still remains. Continuity of care is of vital importance, especially to many of the seriously mentally ill population. With the advent of telemedicine, a psychiatrist may be able to live in a less remote community and to provide services to a more isolated area. This has been the case with Apache County. For other communities experiencing staff shortages, NARBHA Net has increased the availability of psychiatric care as physicians from some Service Area Agencies have provided medical coverage to others. Addressing professional isolation has also been helpful for physician continuity. Northern Arizona psychiatrists meet monthly over NARBHA Net to discuss clinical and administrative issues. CME opportunities also increase physician satisfaction and retention.

Quality of Care

There is an evolving literature regarding the quality of telemedical care. Zarate et al. (1997) began looking at this issue in 1997. They compared telemedicine against face-to-face evaluations in the assessment of schizophrenia and found the former to be as reliable as the latter for global severity and positive symptoms. However, they did find that a higher bandwidth was required to assess negative symptoms. NARBHA Net operates on a bandwidth even higher than the highest that Zarate et al. studied.

NARBHA has also evaluated quality by comparing the outcomes of its telemedicine clients in Apache County with those of all its clients in northern Arizona. These studies can be subject to overinterpretation because of the relatively small number of clients served in Apache County. Medication costs and hospitalization rates for 1997 through mid-2000 were gathered for children and adult populations, and there were no significant differences between telemedicine clients and clients overall.

NARBHA initially made the assumption that the use of telemedicine would result in increased hospitalization rates. Because the psychiatrist would not be assessing the client in person, it was thought that the accuracy of the assessment would be compromised and the threshold for hospitalization would be lower. This has not been the case. In 1996, the year before the telemedicine system was implemented, the hospitalization rate in Apache County was 11.2 per 1,000 clients per month. In 1997, the first full year of utilizing only telemedicine, the rate actually went down to 7.7. However, these numbers shouldn't be overinterpreted, because there were many different variables involved. The practice styles of the two different psychiatrists may have been a more significant determinant of the hospitalization rate than their use of telemedicine. In addition, the increased use of atypical antipsychotics and other medication innovations were important during this time. Crisis workers on call also changed, and an increased degree of comfort with emergency situations may have decreased hospitalization rates. With the small absolute number of hospitalizations, hospitalization rates fluctuate wildly and are difficult to study. However, despite the poor data quality, these results give us a snapshot of inpatient utilization and support the hypothesis that telemedicine practice is within the standard of care in Northern Arizona, without overutilization or gross underutilization of inpatient facilities.

Dr. Gibson (who, as mentioned earlier, provides psychiatric services for the Apache County clinics over NARBHA Net) has been pleasantly surprised at the ease with which she can use the Abnormal Involuntary Movement Scale (AIMS) to track the severity of extrapyramidal side effects induced by antipsychotic medications. As discussed previously, the AIMS involves examination of gait, posture, and gross motor movements, but also looks for fine tremors of the face, tongue, and hands. By utilizing the zoom capabilities, Dr. Gibson subjectively feels that she is able to perform an examination that is equivalent and in some ways superior to an examination in person. By zooming in, the entire television screen can be filled with a closeup of the tongue or hand, and she can search for tremors without invading the patient's personal space. NARBHA is now collaborating with the University of Arizona to study the sensitivity of the AIMS using videoconferencing more objectively.

Subjectively, there are times when Dr. Gibson feels unable to assess a client adequately over NARBHA Net. When this occurs, she refers the client to his or her therapist, primary care physician, or an inpatient facility. However, these instances are rare. Dr. Gibson has also been able to use the telemedicine system to refine the emphasis of the Apache County clinics on a team treatment model. NARBHA policy requires a case manager or therapist to be with the client while videoconferencing with the psychiatrist (although exceptions can be made). Having all members of the treatment team present has been an ideal that was seldom achieved prior to NARBHA Net. The entire clinical staff in Apache County feels that the delivery of clinical care has been improved by this team treatment model and that is more than compensates for any disadvantages for the psychiatrist.

Costs and Savings

Cost is arguably the major impediment to the implementation of a successful telemedicine program. NARBHA, like most telemedicine programs, had an outside grant to get started. NARBHA minimizes cost by employing used equipment, piggybacking T1 lines, and using T1 lines for multiple purposes where feasible. However, we have a high equipment and line standard that drives up our cost. In 1998–1999, NARBHA's expenditures for 14 telemedicine sites, telecommunication costs, salaries, depreciation, and maintenance were $778,994. Approximately $133,000 of that will ultimately be reimbursed by the Universal Service Fund program.

However, there are also significant cost and time savings. During this same 1998–1999 period, 6,572 hours of staff travel time, 347,039 miles of staff travel, and $107,582 of staff travel reimbursement were saved.

Because over 90% of the clients seen by NARBHA Service Area Agencies are funded through the State of Arizona or through Arizona's Medicaid program, there are few reimbursement issues, although Medicare cannot be billed. Private insurers initially denied some payments, but individually contacting them, providing them with articles about telemedicine, and posing questions to them such as "Would you rather have your member drive 7 hours?" have resulted in reimbursement. This reimbursement has been at the same rate as reimbursements for psychiatrist bills for in-person evaluations, but there has been no reimbursement for the time spent by the social worker or the case manager who is on site with the client.

Acceptance

Feedback has been overwhelmingly positive from both clients and staff. Although some clients initially may have had reservations, no clients have refused telemedicine services. Staff and client satisfaction surveys were conducted for the first 3 years of the program, and overall acceptance of videoconferencing as a means to deliver clinical services and to conduct training and educational activities and administrative meetings was high among both staff and clients. Surveys were periodically reviewed and changed as the program developed and certain issues arose or became unimportant. One of the most interesting findings was that clients tended to rate picture quality, sound quality, and comfort with the equipment significantly higher than staff did.

By the second quarter of 1999, 3 years into the program, it was becoming very apparent from the survey responses that both staff and clients were tired of completing surveys about their level of satisfaction. Ironically, several staff members and clients responded on their surveys that continually having to fill out the surveys was leading them to become dissatisfied with the system.

Comments from 1998 and 1999 client satisfaction surveys included:

- She just talks to me like a normal person.
- I'm getting better. It gets easier every time.
- I like it that my family can be present.
- I felt comfortable, and the doctor gave my son the time he needed to explain his feelings.
- Don't change a thing! I like her [the doctor] being her!
- Coming here has made a difference in me and my children because I'm able to get medication and counseling.
- This is a great way to cover the miles for we that are remote.
- I think the services are long overdue for this area. Thank you.
- I appreciate and like what this facility is doing for me, my children even benefit from me doing better from coming to this site, it was different at first, but now more comfortable, it seems to be more effective.

Acceptance and thus utilization of NARBHA Net have grown so high that problems are now arising because of the heavy demand. NARBHA policy is that clinical activities are the highest priority and other videoconferences have to be bumped from the schedule if a clinical need arises.

Clinical Care Principles

Telepsychiatry and Human Interaction

The basic clinical challenge for the health care provider is to provide the highest-quality health care, regardless of the medium. For the psychiatrist, providing this care requires the ability to communicate with the patient. Evaluating and diagnosing a patient's mental status needs historical information that can be conveyed verbally or in writing. Nonverbal, visual cues enhance assessment of the current emotional state and mental status. For the actual provision of care, the psychiatrist must win the trust of the patient so that treatment recommendations can be discussed and informed consent obtained. The psychiatrist must convey empathy and understanding to establish and continually build on this relationship. There is a general concern that the provision of psychiatric services over a videoconferencing system will result in a loss of human interaction, which will hinder quality therapeutic care. NARBHA psychiatrists are asked, "How can you really talk to someone over a machine?" For the clinics in Apache County, this issue was especially prominent. The psychiatrist who had been practicing there prior to the introduction of telemedicine was an integral, vital part of the community. As is the case with many rural physicians, she saw clients out and about town on a daily basis and was highly visible and involved in local life. Clients knew where she lived, brought her homemade cookies, sought her out for consultations in the grocery store, and called her at home. To replace this very warm and human presence with a psychiatrist on a machine was a frightening prospect for the clinic staff and the clients, and a considerable challenge for the new "telepsychiatrist."

The underlying challenge was to move beyond the technical (the cameras and the touchpads) to the human (the trusting doctor–patient and colleague–colleague relationships that facilitate ongoing treatment). Both clients and staff at the two clinics in Apache County have felt that the new system for delivery of care has far exceeded their initial negative expectations. Some of the success can be attributed to the high quality of transmission that NARBHA elected to provide. Having a live, interactive system with no distortion minimizes reminders that the interaction is being moderated by machines. Clients frequently comment that during their initial evaluation, they "forgot" it was telemedicine.

Through experience, NARBHA has also found other ways to help staff and clients "forget the machine." Picture-within-picture or a second monitor at the client's site was quickly eliminated because it was found to be extremely distracting and sometimes distressing for clients to watch themselves ("I look terrible," "I'm so fat"). Zooming the camera in on the psychiatrist (to show mostly her head and shoulders) makes the picture as close to life sized and therefore as lifelike as possible. Having the case manager or therapist present helps to diminish the client's anxiety. Staff also ensure that the telemedicine room is clearly marked "in use," so that there are no interruptions or breaches of confidentiality. Prior to the initial interaction, the client is shown the psychiatrist's site by moving the camera around. This helps the client visualize the setting in which the psychiatrist is located, and reassures the client that others are not observing the session.

Developing rapport in a videoconference interaction requires the same skills as an interaction in person. Use of appropriate body language and facial expression facilitate projection of personality and professional demeanor. Eye contact is a primary mode of communication in our society. Attention to camera angles creates the illusion of direct eye contact (as discussed by Burgiss, Smith, Dimmick, and Welsh, 1998). The camera angles need to be as natural as possible. It doesn't work for the client to look at the psychiatrist's forehead or chin, and the psychiatrist's gaze must appear to rest on the client (i.e., be on the camera rather than on the monitor) to better approximate direct eye contact.

Confidentiality is essential in psychiatric practice, and clients are carefully reassured as to the security of their communication with the psychiatrist (as described in this chapter's appendices). This issue is discussed prior to and reinforced during the initial psychiatric evaluation. A consent to participate in telemedicine (see the appendices) is also signed prior to the first session. Although administrative videoconferences are videotaped, videotaping of clinical sessions is not routinely done because it might present a significant impediment to maintaining clients' trust and their confidence that their confidentiality will be vigorously protected. An exception is made, with their informed consent, for clients with tardive dyskinesia, who are taped to document the course of their symptoms over time and to research the use of telemedicine to evaluate these subtle movements.

Technical difficulties are always a problem when dealing with machines. The telemedicine system sometimes is subject to minor distortions on stormy days (in Arizona, during the 6-week summer monsoon season). They can interfere with the therapeutic relationship and serve as a reminder that there are indeed 180 miles and a machine separating the client from the psychiatrist. Most clients have experienced this at least once and have learned to laugh and to go on with the session. Minor distortions are more of a problem with a new client, during the crucial initial period of building rapport, instilling trust, and establishing a therapeutic alliance. There have been several technical "disasters" in which the entire T1 phone line went down and telemedicine services were unavailable for an entire day. To compound the problem, many clients in Apache County do not have a home telephone and cannot be contacted at the last minute to reschedule their appointments. NARBHA minimizes the impact of a sudden unavailability of the telemedicine system by having clients meet with their therapist or case manager in person and the psychiatrist by telephone. Fortunately, such technical disasters have been rare, and their frequency has significantly diminished over time.

Transference, Countertransference, and Boundaries

Psychiatrists are attentive to transference and countertransference, the doctor–patient relationship, and boundaries. All are clearly affected by the insertion of technology between the psychiatrist and the patient. To NARBHA's surprise, some of these effects have been very positive. Clients have been more respectful of appointment times, viewing the telemedicine session as more "professional" than traditional in-person sessions. The physician appointment times have become more encapsulated, with the entire clinic staff working to keep the psychiatrist "on time." Clients express pride in having a "big city" doctor and in being on the cutting edge of technology and health care delivery. The physical distance from the psychiatrist helps to focus the client on the local treatment team and therapy as opposed to the psychiatrist and medications. This subtle shift also emphasizes the client's own responsibility to work on problems rather than seeking quick fixes (although that certainly still occurs).

Different patient populations have varying responses to their initial telemedicine experience. Children tend to be very comfortable with technology (especially computers and TV) and exhibit very little anxiety. They even play telemedicine jokes, like hiding under the table where the camera can't see, or singing into the microphone. Elderly clients tend to be uncomfortable with the technology, as do adults with social phobias, posttraumatic stress disorders, and other anxiety disorders. There were some attempts early on to stratify patients based on their ability to see the psychiatrist in person in Flagstaff, but it was decided that all patients, regardless of diagnosis or payor type, would be seen in the same manner, over NARBHA Net.

Some sites have reported that psychotic, particularly schizophrenic, patients feel "safer" in telemedicine sessions. In general, our experience has been mixed. Very paranoid, delusional patients can also be more suspicious of the technology and incorporate it into an existing delusional system, but this has been rare. One patient with poor interpersonal skills did indeed seem more comfortable with the "distance" of telemedicine. But in general, across diagnoses, there is an initial wariness or anxiety that is replaced over time with acceptance.

Perhaps some of our success is due to the fact that we don't apologize for this system. In fact, we view it as an overwhelmingly positive solution to the challenge of delivering care to a historically underserved population. Besides, everyone—regardless of age, diagnosis, or severity of impairment—is seen over NARBHA Net. Clients seldom even comment on the system anymore. It is simply how we do business.

References

Burgiss, S. G., Smith, G. T., Dimmick, S. L., & Welsh, T. S. (1998, August). Improving telepresence during consultations. *Telemedicine Today, 6*(4), 14–15.

Zarate, C. A., Weinstock, L., Cukor, P., Morabito, C., Leahy, L., Burns, C., & Baer, L. (1997). Applicability of telemedicine for assessing patients with schizophrenia: Acceptance and reliability. *Journal of Clinical Psychiatry, 58*, 22–25.

Appendices

Technical Description

Currently, there are 14 northern Arizona sites connected by private, dedicated T1 phone lines. There is also the capacity for two Primary Rate Interface connections to the outside world and full T1 lines to the Community Partnership of Southern Arizona network (which includes Behavioral Health Services), the single Pinal Gila Regional Behavioral Health Association site, and the University of Arizona Telemedicine Program. All 14 of the NARBHA Net sites have internal inverse multiplexer connections; the University of Arizona site has a direct connection. At the hub in Flagstaff, a Network Equipment Technologies IDNX 90 PrimeVideo Switching System allows private video and data network connections and is configured for both on- and off-network video dial-up capability. Dedicated T1 phone lines from the remote locations connect from local telecommunication carriers into the hub through Adtran TSU channel service units, which carry those 24 channels into the IDNX 90, where they are then split out, dedicating eight channels for video, one for control and signaling information (the D-channel), and the remaining 15 for data and voice applications. The eight video channels and the one D-channel are then fed into a multipoint conferencing unit (MCU) switching device that interconnects H.320 compliant conference systems. This MCU permits any combination of the 14 sites and up to two outside agencies (e.g., hospitals, universities, or out-of-state clinics) to participate in videoconferences.

Each remote site is equipped with an Adtran TSU, which accepts the other end of the T1 line from Flagstaff and feeds into the router, where those 24 channels are split out into video, data, or voice. The majority of the video equipment is still Compression Laboratories, Inc., Radiance 8750s and 8775s, with one VTEL TC2000. These room videoconferencing units are all equipped with a television monitor and an open PC system that codes analog signals into digital signals for transmission and decodes them for reception, allowing two-way, live video transactions.

The dedicated T1 network is a permanent, nonswitched ("nailed-up") connection between the NARBHA sites, leased by the sites from various telecommunication carriers, which allows 24 hour/day, 7 day/week full T1 service. Only those sites directly physically hooked into the private network have access to it.

Through the Primary Rate Interface (PRI), an outside entity could enter into a NARBHA videoconference. PRI access to NARBHA's video network is enabled using a Teleos network access device that routes video calls from outside entities into the NARBHA network through the NARBHA MCU. This network connection works similarly to the way the dedicated T1 lines are connected to the network MCU through the Adtran TSUs. Confidentiality is assured; if an outside entity wants to participate in one of NARBHA's videoconferences, it must ask the conference manager to set that specific meeting up to allow that site in. In other words, an outside caller cannot just call in and successfully connect. A one-time dial-in number (based on the channels available at the time of the call) and the video and audio protocols, transmission rate, and so on, of the particular videoconference are required.

In many locations around the country, telecommunication carriers offer customers the option to lease fractional T1 lines or ISDN lines instead of full point-to-point 1.54 mbps T1 paths. Unfortunately for the NARBHA budget, in rural Arizona, this was not an option. Full point-to-point T1 paths were the only means of ensuring total confidentiality.

Because a 512 kbps videoconference utilizes slightly less than half of a T1 line, there was additional bandwidth available for use. When possible, NARBHA "piggybacks" two remote sites on one T1 line to the hub in Flagstaff to make better use of those lines. For example, a T1 line originates in Springerville, is directed to St. Johns, and terminates at the hub in Flagstaff. The T1 line from St. Johns to Flagstaff has the capacity to carry two videoconferences, one between St. Johns and Flagstaff and another between Springerville and Flagstaff, making use of 18 (8 video and one D- each) of the 24 channels on that T1. This avoids having to pay for a separate full T1 line from from St. Johns to Flagstaff. St. Johns piggybacks onto the Springerville line. To further maximize the use of this T1 line, the six remaining channels are configured for transmitting data and, in some cases, voice, thus saving on long-distance telephone calls.

Consent to Participate in Telemedicine

NARBHA Net

Consent to Participate

I, _____, have been asked to participate as a client on the NARBHA Net telemedicine network. I will be receiving health care services through interactive video equipment. I understand the use of video equipment is a new method of health care delivery. I understand that, at this time, there are no known risks involved with receiving my care in this way.

I understand the equipment will be shown to me and I will get to see how it works before I receive any services. I understand my participation in this is totally voluntary and I may decide to quit at any time. My privacy and confidentiality will be protected at all times. When I am receiving services over the video, I can see who is in the room at the other site.

I give my consent to receive services over the videoconferencing equipment. I understand the services I receive will become part of my treatment record at the clinic. I understand the health care providers at both sites will have access to any relevant medical information about me including any psychiatric and/or psychological information, alcohol and/or drug abuse, and mental health records.

I have read this document and I hereby consent to participate in NARBHA Net under the terms described above. I understand this document will become a part of my medical record.

_____   _____
Client Signature   Date

_____
Witness Signature

The above release is given on behalf of _____because the client is a minor or has been determined to be incompetent to give medical consent.

_____

Parent or Legal Guardian Signature   Date

_____

Relationship to Client

_____

Witness Signature

5

Chat Room Therapy

Gary S. Stofle

OVER THE PAST SEVERAL years, mental health professionals have debated
the possibility of online psychotherapy. Whether in opposition to or support
of the practice, professionals have shared the same concerns: the lack of research, therapist competency, the lack of nonverbal (visual and auditory) cues,
uncertainty regarding client age and identity, potential problems with confidentiality, national and international oversight and licensure issues, and the
suicidal client (Barak, 1999; Childress, 1998; Gross, 2000; Hartwell-Walker,
2000; Holmes, 1997; Stofle, 1997; Suler, 2000). This chapter discusses these
concerns in the context of the provision of therapy in a chat room. Transcripts
of chat sessions demonstrate the range of possibilities inherent in chat room
therapy. Examples from single-session, short-term, and long-term treatment
illustrate how chat room therapy varies in length and is helpful in different
circumstances, much like therapy in person.

General Issues in Chat Room Therapy

Lack of Research

Little research exists regarding the provision of therapy in a chat room. Barak
(1999) compared group therapy in a chat room to group therapy in person
and used a nontherapy group as a control. Although the results were cau-
tiously interpreted, both the chat room therapy and the therapy in person
showed a "small, statistically insignificant positive improvement in participants' self-image, social relations, and well-being, with a trend in favor of

the virtual group" (Barak, 1999, p. 1). The International Society of Mental Health Online (www.ismho.org) conducted a clinical case study group (www.ismho.org/ccsg) that included chat room therapy as one of the case studies. Although hypotheses concerning the provision of e-therapy services in general have been developed from these case studies, no coherent and overarching theory of therapy in a chat room has resulted (Suler & Fenichel, 2000).

Despite the lack of research and theory regarding e-therapy, it is practiced every day and is "here to stay" (Grohol, 1997, p. 6). Online clinics have been created to provide therapists with secure areas where they can meet with clients via chat or e-mail (see, e.g., www.helphorizons.com). eTherapy.com had an electronic tutorial for new therapists as a part of an orientation to practice on their Web site (S. Mankita, personal communication, August 6, 2000). A number of therapists have created Web pages advertising their e-therapy services. Metanoia.org (www.metanoia.org) is a consumer-run Web site that— as a public service—lists, rates, and links to e-therapists, some of whom offer therapy using chat rooms. It has been anticipated that more and more online clinics will open, some of which will be sponsored by managed care companies (Wylie, 2000).

Therapist Competency

Is a therapist who is competent in person necessarily competent online? No, but experience and training in conducting therapy in person are essential to be able to conduct therapy competently online (International Society of Mental Health Online & Psychiatric Society of Informatics, 2000; Stofle, 1997).

The efficacy of psychotherapy in person is widely accepted. "The Efficacy of Psychotherapy" (www.apa.org/practice/peff.html), by the American Psychological Association, cites extensive research that clearly indicates the efficacy of different modalities of psychotherapy. A *Consumer Reports* survey, reportedly the largest single study of therapy as it is actually practiced, clearly demonstrated the effectiveness of psychotherapy (Seligman, 1995).

Part of being competent is applying appropriate treatments and interventions to the issues that the client presents (Sanderson & Woody, 1995). Clients' issues are the same, whether at brick-and-mortar or online clinics. Treatment goals are also the same. The paradigms for understanding clients and their issues do not change when practicing online; rather, the methods of intervention must be adapted to fit the methods of communication. In addition to experience and competency providing therapy in person, chat room therapists must possess online comfort and savvy, typing ability, and skill in using text to communicate—both to understand the client and to make themselves understood to the client.

Lack of Nonverbals

A number of authors have stated emphatically that therapy is impossible online because of the lack of nonverbals (e.g., Childress, 1998; Holmes, n. d.). The nonverbal information obtained when meeting with a client in person is valuable in assessing and working with him or her. A chat room therapist cannot compare what the client says against his or her body movements, dress, voice inflection, and degree of tenseness or relaxation, nor use that information to help the client learn more about himself or herself. Neither can the chat room therapist use a smile and a warm handshake to help engage the client in the treatment process. This might appear to be a barrier to effective and ethical chat room therapy.

How can a therapeutic relationship be developed using only text? A concept that helps clarify this is called "presence" (Fink, 1999; Lombard & Ditton, 1997). Presence is the perception that a video- or computer-mediated experience is not actually mediated. During a chat session, the therapist and the client each may feel as though the other is physically present. That feeling of presence is contributed to by all of the ways each person presents in that chat room at that moment in time. This includes screen or chat name, font style, typing speed, interaction tempo, verbosity, use of colloquialisms and emoticons, and spelling and grammar. Another term for this might be *nontextuals*, that is, everything other than the words themselves. Although not all of these factors are specifically evaluated while online, many can be assessed through a review of the transcript, and they all add to the feeling of presence.

A sensitive therapist can know a client's baseline chat room demeanor and notice deviations from it. For example, a therapist and client met as scheduled in a chat room for their weekly session. Within minutes, the therapist sensed that something was different. He even wondered if the person he was working with was actually his client. He quickly confronted the client, and she revealed she had been drinking prior to the session. The therapist ended the session and rescheduled it. The client did not slur her typing, but something was off. It is essential for the chat room therapist to have sensitivity to nontextuals.

Client Identity

The issue of client identity is of utmost concern for online therapists (Childress, 1998; Gross, 2000). In face-to-face therapy, we take for granted that people who call and show up for an appointment are who they say they are—I've never said, "Let's see some ID" before going into an intake session. In a chat room, however, all that's available is a screen name and possibly a profile on the site. Questions immediately come to mind: Is this person a minor? Does this person indeed have the characteristics he or she reports? How can I work with a person who won't reveal basic demographic information about himself or herself?

Could an adolescent pose as an adult and seek therapy services? Yes, I believe it could be done, at least in the short term. (No matter how distracted a parent might be, eventually charges on a credit card would be noticed.) But why would an adolescent do that? My experience in therapy is that it's not something that one would do for a "kick": It's just too much hard work. If a young person posed as an adult to participate in therapy for a "kick," that would, to me, represent a significant problem by itself (and one that could not be addressed until the client's true identity were discovered).

I've received a number of "instant messages" over the years from adolescents asking for help. All were completely open about their age, and I referred each to local, face-to-face treatment or self-help, such as school counselors or Alateen.

Therapists can choose whom they serve. The more conservative approach is to ask for complete demographic information from a prospective client and to verify the information prior to beginning therapy. Although it is risky to provide services to clients who refuse to identify themselves, some therapists choose to do so because of their ethical commitment to providing services to clients who may not otherwise participate in therapy.

Confidentiality

Confidentiality is an integral component of every ethical code for human service workers. In order for a client to open up to a therapist, the client has to have a sense that what he or she says will not be revealed to anyone else without his or her permission. Childress (1998) talked about four ways that the confidentiality of e-therapy communications is at risk: during transmission, while saved on the therapist's computer, while saved on the client's computer, and after being subpoenaed. E-mail can be intercepted during transmission because the Internet relies on copying information in order to send it. Clinical data stored on either the therapist's or the client's end, if not password protected, is available to anyone who has access to that computer. Also, if the client e-mails the therapist from work, that e-mail is the property of and may be legally read by the client's employer. In addition, because courts have not decided whether e-mail between a therapist and a client is privileged information, it may be subject to subpoena.

Some professionals note that confidentiality in face-to-face therapy is not secure either. Shulman (2000) wrote that confidentiality has been lost because managed care requires that, every so many sessions, the therapist send a report "detailing your private discussions." Ainsworth (n.d.) ventured that "talking to a therapist online is probably as safe as talking to one in person. Both are very confidential, and neither is 100% perfect." Grohol (1999) compared the potential risk of breaches of confidentiality online and in person: "While the on-line world does indeed offer its fair share of risks to a client's confidentiality and privacy, it is not readily apparent that these risks are significantly or inherently greater than similar risks already taken in real-world therapy sessions."

Oversight and Licensure

Concern has been expressed about the provision of services to a client who lives in a state in which the therapist is not licensed to practice (Childress, 1998; Gross, 2000; Holmes, 1997). The California Telemedicine Development Act of 1996 "restricts California telemedicine services to practioniers licensed in California. This means we cannot communicate electronically as primary care providers with clients/patients outside of our state" (Maheu, 1999).

E-therapy gives clients the opportunity to receive expert treatment that may not be available to them in person. Geographical location is not an issue. A client who is experiencing depression, for example, and is willing and able to be treated online can search the World Wide Web and find an expert to consult. A client in Connecticut can get help for self-esteem issues from a therapist in Oregon. Should the therapist in Oregon be licensed in Connecticut? As treatment professionals who are participating in the development of ethical codes and legislation regarding e-therapy, we need to be mindful not to recreate barriers to treatment that the Internet has eliminated.

The Suicidal Client

This important issue is often discussed in relation to e-therapy. The scenario is this: You begin a counseling relationship with a client who is unwilling to provide any demographic information about himself or herself. You correspond by e-mail (or chat), and then one day you receive the following e-mail: "That's it! I'm outta here. I'm going to kill myself today. I have the means to do it. Thanks for everything." If this threat were made while meeting in person, the therapist would be able to facilitate the client's getting to a hospital, where he or she would be safe.

The issue is one of powerlessness. What can you do when there is nothing you can do? The better comparison would be receiving a suicide e-mail from a client whose location you've never known versus receiving a suicide voice mail from a client who, so as not to be stopped, is going to a location you don't know. In both cases, you are powerless.

Being seen in person by a helping professional often does not deter a suicidal client. An NIMH study reported that 70% of elderly people who commit suicide visit their family doctors within a month prior to their suicide, and 39% have a medical encounter within a week prior to killing themselves (Ohio Department of Rehabilitation, n.d.). We need to acknowledge our powerlessness with clients who are fully determined to commit suicide.

As mentioned earlier, therapists need to make decisions regarding whom we will treat online and under what circumstances we will treat them. Most therapists will not treat an acutely suicidal client online because such clients need a more intensive level of care for their own protection. E-therapy can be conceptualized as a level of care that is indicated for people with certain problems or issues. A client's issues and problems must be assessed initially, and an appropriate level of care then advised. If the client's needs change and a different level of care is required, the therapist must make appropriate recommendations. If a face-to-face therapy client becomes suicidal, the therapist refers the client for a psychiatric evaluation and possible hospitalization. The same process applies to e-therapy clients.

Table 5.1 looks at different levels of care and indicates where e-therapy fits. The need for a specific level of care is determined by client functioning along several dimensions, one of which is suicidality.

Practical Issues in Chat Room Therapy

There are practical issues and potential problems related to the provision of therapy in a chat room. Although it is beyond the scope of this chapter to provide an in-depth exploration of all of the potential issues, several of importance are discussed here.

No Obvious Client

The "no obvious client" problem can occur when the therapist is working online with a client while in the physical presence of others. Colleagues at the office or family members at home can distract the therapist because they are unaware that the therapist is in the middle of an online session. In contast to

TABLE 5.1
Levels of Care

	SUICIDALITY/ HOMICIDALITY	RELATIONSHIPS WITH OTHERS
Level 5: Outpatient therapy in person or online	Has occasional passive suicidal ideation or no suicidal thoughts. Has no homicidal thoughts.	Has problems in relationships that cause some distress (e.g., has difficulty with openness and intimacy, blames others).
Level 4: Intensive outpatient therapy in person or online	Has persistent passive suicidal ideation. Can contract for safety. Has angry feelings toward others with no plan or intent to act them out.	Has problems in relationships that cause great distress.
Level 3: Day treatment	Same as level 4.	Has intense, unstable relationships.
Level 2: Partial hospitalization	Same as level 4.	Same as level 3.
Level 1: Inpatient hospitalization*	Is acutely suicidal or acutely homicidal.	Avoids relationships.

*May not need inpatient treatment. All Level 1 issues need, at minimum, a psychiatric evaluation to determine the appropriate level of care.
Adapted, with permission, from Stofle (2001).

sessions in person, there is no obvious client. In order to remain undisturbed, therapists need to find ways to alert those around them when they are in a chat room session.

No Oversight by the Client

In chat room therapy, the client does not observe the therapist's behavior, which increases the potential for the therapist to be distracted. Because the client is not watching, the therapist is free to behave in ways that would not be appropriate otherwise (e.g., to look out the window or to turn on the stereo). The potential for self-distraction is enormous exactly when the therapist needs to be more rather than less focused. It takes an extraordinary amount of concentration to provide therapy in a chat room. The therapist needs to have an acute sense of timing to be able to respond in a manner

TABLE 5.1
(continued)

PARTICIPATION IN THE WORLD	REALITY TESTING	FEELINGS/ISSUES
Participates actively in the world.	Has erroneous beliefs about self (e.g., doesn't see self as worthwhile, has self-esteem problems).	Lacks feelings, management skills. Has ongoing uncomfortable feelings.
Has some difficulty with active participation in the world.	Has erroneous beliefs about the world that cause temporary impairment.	Has feelings that cause great distress.
Participates in the world only with family, a few friends, or an inappropriate support system.	Has chronic problems with disordered thinking.	Has feelings that interfere with some aspects of life.
Is isolated from the world except for contact with the therapist.	Has disordered thinking that interferes with multiple aspects of life.	Has feelings that interfere with multiple aspects of life.
Is isolated from the world.	Has disordered thinking that impairs basic functioning.	Has feelings that impair basic functioning.

that reveals the therapist's attentiveness and knowledge of the issues being presented. For example, when the therapist poses a question to the client, the therapist has to start an internal timer. If the client doesn't respond within an appropriate period of time, a follow-up question needs to be asked.

The most direct way to deal with this "oversight" issue is to discuss it with the client in the first session. In the examples that follow this section, that was not done. However, in subsequent chat room therapy cases, I have always talked to the client about this issue and asked the client about his or her typing speed, comfort and experience in chat rooms, and so on.

Disrupted Turn Adjacency

In chat interactions, "messages are not necessarily addressed in the order they are received" (S. Mankita, personal communication, August 6, 2000). Although this is much more of an issue in a group chat than in a chat between two people, it may present a problem when beginning to work with a client. This was the case with Clients A and B, in large part because of the newness of the chat room therapy process for both the author and the clients and the author's unfamiliarity with these clients' communication styles. It can be distracting when the therapist moves on to another issue only to find the client needs to discuss the previous issue further. Disrupted turn adjacency was less of an issue with Client C. We had worked together for a period of time before that session, and so we each had a good sense of the other's timing and communication tempo. The solution to this problem is for the therapist to develop a very good sense of the style and rhythm of the client's communication and to adjust his or her interventions accordingly.

Examples of Chat Room Therapy

The transcripts that follow are from the chat room therapy practice I conducted between December 1996 and June 1999. Several clients found my practice by viewing my profile on America Online (AOL). A profile can be created for every screen name on AOL, and can contain the following information: real name, location, gender, marital status, hobbies, computers, occupation, and personal quote. AOL members use their profiles to communicate a variety of information. At one point, I mentioned in my profile that I was a therapist who worked with adult children of alcoholics; I subsequently received several referrals.

The chat sessions were conducted on AOL. Private chat rooms were easily created using an AOL "buddy list." No additional hardware or software was required to create or participate in chat rooms, only AOL membership. For ongoing clients, chat sessions were held weekly for 50 to 60 minutes. Fees were based upon a sliding scale. For these sessions, payments were made by check ahead of time. For subsequent ones, I have successfully used PayPal (www.paypal.com).

A typical chat session would begin like this: The client would sign on to AOL, and I would send him or her an instant message saying something like, "Hi! Are you ready to start the session?" I would then create a private chat room using the standard AOL software. The room name would be based on my screen name and a randomly generated number. When the client was ready, I would send him or her an invitation to join me. All the client would have to do was click the "Go" button on the chat room invitation, and he or she would be in the chat room.

To preserve the feel of the interactions, these transcripts have only been edited slightly. The ellipses were part of the dialogue and do not indicate omissions. Consecutive chat messages by one person have been condensed for readability. Some information has been changed to protect client confidentiality.

Single-Session Chat Room Triage and Referral

Client A contacted me, asking to meet and to discuss problems in her life. She found me through my profile on AOL. I didn't have any clinical information about her, but decided to meet her in a chat room. She was on time for the session and started out by thanking me for being willing to listen to her. Presented here is the transcript of the session, starting about five minutes after the session began.

[Client A]: growing up my uncle sexually molested me & my sister, she has no feelings about it

[Therapist]: have you been in treatment before about these issues?

then my father always called me all different kinds of "fat" names. i went to the eap program offered thru my work but just didn't feel like it helped

hmmm . . . often it's not enough. so go on.

my father was an alcoholic, still is, I have nothing to do with him. he would call me every name there was, hit me in front of my friends if i didn't get up & get him another beer. Now everything he used to say to me I realize is affecting me in everything I do

yes.

I can't really talk to anyone in my family. Me & my sister fight about it constantly because

have you been to ACOA [Adult Children of Alcoholics] meetings?

I got the schedule & was thinking of going tonight. There's a meeting down the street from me but I've never been

I'm sorry I interrupted you.

oh that's ok it's just my sister thinks my father did no wrong. It didn't have an effect on her so she thinks I'm stupid & a b**ch for feeling the way I do. my mom acts like she could care less. Also it's hard for me to find any friends to talk to about it because I don't trust anyone

what is your situation now? do you live with your family?

no. I live by myself

same town as your family?

about 45 minutes away from each other

how old are you?

Sometimes I feel like it's not far enough away. I'm 27

are you working?

yes sir

Gary . . . :o)

sorry

it's ok. that's right—you said you went through your EAP. how long ago was that?

It was about 6 or 7 months ago

ok. I need to ask you whether or not you've thought of hurting yourself. in the past, or right now.

Here lately all of the time. I'm just so tired of feeling the way I do

do you have a plan for how you would hurt yourself?

Never being able to please my parents, even now. Each time I think about it I always think of pills

do you have pills now?

none that I think would really do any harm

good. you need to understand that if you are thinking about hurting yourself, you need to see someone in person . . . it's much safer than online. the person can physically help you be safe.

I just don't know who to turn to

and that's the most important thing. what town do you live in?

[She gives her city and state.] there's a local place but then I'm afraid they will tell my work

Is it a treatment center?

& I will get into trouble for trying to take any time off. yes. they treat alco-holics, depression

if you are thinking about hurting yourself, getting in trouble at work is not the biggest problem. they can't release information to your employer without your permission.

I try to tell myself that they can't fire me for something like that but they won't let us take any time off

you are right . . . it's against the law. what hours do you work?

right now we've been working from 6am–8pm & it's hard to find the time to see someone in person

Saturdays as well?

he told us starting this Saturday we have to start working Saturdays also but I'm not sure of the hours on Saturdays

maybe you could call the treatment center and see if they have hours later in the evening.

i can try that

good . . . if you get to the point where you don't think about hurting yourself then we can deal with at least some of these issues online.

ok

issues about self esteem, feelings management, dealing with family issues.

alright

you hit the nail on the head when you said how your father and family treated you affects how you look at yourself now.

if anyone shows interest in me I find all kinds of faults in them because I feel like I'm not worth someone actually liking me

at the same time, I bet you are very kind towards others.

I always do for others before myself. I can't seem to say no to anyone. especially when my mom always wants to borrow money, then I end up resenting her for always asking me after she's blown hers

and you get mad at yourself as well, heh?

if i get the courage to tell her no she ends up mad at me & won't speak to me. yes i do

so then you give in and give her what she wants.

yes even if it leaves me without any until I get paid again

that's not fair to you.

no but at least it keeps her happy & speaking to me

the work ahead for you boils down to one sentence: you need to learn how to take better care of yourself.

I know but just don't know how

that's what treatment is about.

without causing so many other problems

you need to hear there will be some problems as you get better (just like there are problems right now).

I've seen that with the way my sister acts towards me now since I said everything has had an effect on me *right.*

I don't understand why it affects me so much but not her. the same things happened to her, except for my father talking to her that way

I don't know. Sometimes people divorce themselves from their feelings. It's a way of coping.

I just feel silly that it's affected me this way after so long. that it didn't bother me sooner instead of later

feelings are real. and no one can tell you that you should or shouldn't feel a certain way.

even though everyone seems to think they can

right . . . they just don't understand how it works.

i guess not

so many people don't understand how to deal with their feelings. yet, it's so much a part of everyone's life. do you have friends?

that's true because I don't know how to deal with the way i feel now either

right.

not really. I have some friends but none that I feel comfortable talking to

we each need at least one person we can talk to on a feelings level.

all of my friends that I felt comfortable enough talking to have gotten married & moved out of state

that must be sad for you.

it is & very hard because I don't really have anyone to get out & do things with & then it's so hard for me to go out & meet new people

are you in a relationship now?

no. just ended one about 2 weeks ago

what happened?

basically what I said earlier. He acted like he liked me for who I was so I tried to find something wrong so I couldn't like him

and you did.

yes. from things like we didn't like the same things, he never wanted to do anything, I ended up always having to pay my way & usually his also, that was the hardest thing for me to deal with

you pay the way for enough people already.

i felt like if i didn't then he wouldn't like me either or i couldn't never get him to do anything

hmmm. what kinds of things do you like to do?

movies, going out to eat, going to hockey games, reading, dancing

do you do those things?

occasionally. i was going to hockey games all of the time, until my mom & stepdad adopted one of the players & started acting like they were more of a family then we were. it made me sick to look at & listen to them so I've got to where I don't hardly go

you must have felt pretty uncomfortable . . .

uncomfortable & like we didn't mean as much anymore because she was always talking & doing for them & not paying any attention to us at all

us meaning you and your sister?

if we asked her a question we had to ask 3 different times for her to even hear us. me & my older sister

it makes sense for you to not want to go.

i've got a question that's kind of away from this

ok go ahead.

I've been having problems with work also, feeling like I don't fit in, it's real hard to get up in the morning & want to go, is it by any chance related to how I've been feeling

there's a good chance it's related.

i've gotten to the point to where I just want to stay inside my apt & not have to deal with anyone

you sound depressed.

is there anything I can do before I end up doing something stupid? I've been looking for a different job, even though I have a really really good job

yes . . . go get an evaluation—that would be the first thing.

from the treatment center?

if they treat depression, yes. Or maybe there's another place close by . . . I don't know the places in your city . . . I'm up in NY.

the center is only about 5 or 10 minutes away from me

that's cool . . . you're worth getting this evaluation. and what you are dealing with can change . . . I've seen it happen with others. you can learn to say no, you can learn to deal with your feelings

i've called them before, about a year ago, but I didn't have the money to go

and the abuse from the past. do you have insurance now?

I've got different insurance now to where I think I only have to pay $100 & then they will pay 80%

that's pretty reasonable nowadays.

but that's only if someone from the EAP refers me to them & they wouldn't do that last time

why not?

they felt like they could help & I felt like they weren't helping at all

did you let them know you had thoughts of hurting yourself?

Yes. They wouldn't switch me to another counselor because I could only go after 5pm & that was the only one that stayed late

that is not acceptable . . . I would go back to the EAP and complain.

I tried changing my hours at work to where one day a week maybe I could go in late & work late but they wouldn't think of it. it's hard to really explain to my supervisor why because she goes & tells all of my co-workers who in turn talk about it among themselves

that's not ethical. what kind of work do you do?

I've confronted her about it but she denies it. accounting

you have to make this happen.

i want to change it & make things better more than anything. I'm so tired of feeling the way I do

your well being is the most important thing. I can understand how you feel tired.

I feel completely drained all of the time

did you know that if you are really feeling like hurting yourself, you can go to the nearest hospital emergency room?

I've thought about moving out of town, changing jobs, a change of scenery but I really don't

they will evaluate you there.

think that's going to change anything. I never knew I could go to the emergency room

right . . . the change has to happen on the inside. most ERs have an on-call psychiatrist.

I never knew that

all do that have a psych unit in the hospital (and many hospitals have a psych unit).

that's something i could check into also

absolutely. do you agree to follow up with what we've been talking about? the EAP, the treatment center?

yes. Thank you for talking with me. I feel better letting some of it out. probably the treatment center & just pay for it myself

do you understand I would like to work with you once you feel a bit more stable?

yes

do you believe that change is possible?

i hope it's possible

:0) hope is good. will you send me an e-mail to let me know what you worked out?

i will

ok... I've enjoyed talking to you tonight... I look forward to hearing from you.

I've enjoyed it also. Thank you

ok... keep in touch...

I will.

good night.

good night. Bye

This transcript illustrates several very important points. Client A was very open from the start of the session. She talked about prior treatment in person, which she felt was ineffective. She also seemed to lack the ability to advocate for herself. She discussed her need to keep the peace by meeting her mother's needs at the expense of her own, then feeling hurt and angry about her behavior (all of which is quite common with adult children of alcoholics). The client also admitted to relatively constant suicidal ideation with a plan, but no current means. When that became apparent, my focus switched from assessment for possible chat room work to referral for treatment in person (although I did discuss the potential of chat room work in the future). She was not opposed to therapy in person, but related an uncomfortable previous experience. My work at that point was to stress the need for follow through despite her previous experience and to remove barriers to her actually seeking treatment in person. Additionally, I informed her of other treatment options that she had not considered in the past.

Client A did follow up with me quite soon after the initial meeting. She went back to the EAP and obtained a referral to the treatment center she had spoken about. She began a course of therapy in person and has not contacted me since for any further chat room work. This was a single-session interaction.

Short-Term Chat Room Therapy

Client B asked to meet so we could discuss online therapy. We met in a chat room and began exploring her issues and goals for treatment. She was a compulsive overeater and had successfully completed a course of therapy in person with a social worker (whom I knew) and a psychiatrist. Since leaving therapy, she had gotten off track and wanted to get back to her personal growth and recovery from her food addiction. This transcript is part of our initial session and begins after she first talked about issues and problems related to her childhood:

[Client B]: A pretty lousy childhood, wouldn't you say? And that was the tip of the iceberg, believe me.

[Therapist]: I understand . . . yes, no child deserves to go through that. children need to be loved and nourished.

It was rough, and I think it weakened me at first, but now strengthened me.

the opposite of your experience.

absolutely.

I want to ask you some questions.

ok

are you on any meds?

No. Dr. Smith had me on luvox for a year, but it did nothing. Just birth control pills now.

ok . . . do you have any thoughts of hurting yourself in any way?

oh no!

very good . . . have you ever?

No, never.

very good. It's important for me to know because of the nature of online work . . . I may never see you . . . and it can be scary for me if you've had a history of suicidal thoughts.

No, never.

that can be a rule-out for online work as well. good.

Well, Gary . . . let me ask you

k

I know I'm a COEater [compulsive over eater], but does that mean I HAVE to deal with this via OA and 12 steps? Every large person who goes to WW [Weight Watchers], or on other plans, is probably COEating as well. Why does it have to be this way for me?

did you have any success with WW?

Temporary. I also did it on my own once and lost 60 lbs. But even OA was temporary.

there are many paths to recovery . . . you have to pick one that ends up being internalized . . . where you live the program even apart from it. you have to find a set of principles that can help you deal with your powerlessness. that's the key to dealing with compulsive behavior.

that sounds like the 12 steps. I have nothing against OA, but I hit some roadblocks there.

let me say something before we go further . . .

ok

as I said in my e-mail, my background is not specifically in eating disorders . . . it's in addictions. Although I have worked with COEs as a part of my addiction work. what do you think about that?

I think addiction and COE are very, very linked.

I don't want to misrepresent myself to you in any way.

I know.

ok

Do you think the substance of food is the same as the substance of say, booze? as far as abstinence is concerned?

yes, but a bit more difficult to deal with because you have to eat something . . . you don't have to drink alcohol.

right.

and many of our celebrations are linked to food

and I'm Italian!!

thanksgiving and so on. wow . . . my wife is Italian . . . pasta every Sunday. I know.

Yes!

the whole family comes over . . . yep. makes it tough.

Practically impossible. It's such comfort food, too.

so, what were the roadblocks in OA?

Well, most of the sponsors I've had, that I've tried to look up to, had more problems than I ever did. There was gossip there, there was judgmental-ness(?). All the things there shouldn't be. I know they say take the best and leave the rest. Plus, there were inconsistencies. Some sponsors allowed certain

principles over personalities.

foods, some didn't. Yes! It just caused me to be resentful and then I'd start lying, and disappear.

do you have more skills now where you can deal with the resentments? more directly?

probably, but when it comes to me and food issues I'm a child!

yes, and you can draw upon the adult self you've developed from all your hard work in therapy to help you.

How do I know if I'm capable of doing this on my own . . . I've failed on my own, failed with help in the past.

oh, I don't think you should start out on your own. that goes against the understanding of powerlessness. you need others to help you now.

Right. I remember in meetings people would screw up when they "took back their will"

or you wouldn't have e-mailed me. that's right.

My therapist was a real tough cookie; Dr. Smith was a softie.

you need someone in the middle. a softie that holds you responsible.

My therapist would torpedo me with questions about food—"why did you break your diet"! Dr. Smith would say, I know this is difficult. Don't beat yourself up.

it is difficult. and you are responsible for the choices you make.

I feel very desperate, Gary.

that can give you the energy to do what you need to do.

The harder I try, the quicker I fail. The less I try, the quicker I fail.

where's the we?

I'm so accomplished in my other areas of my life . . . this really has no rationale. what do you mean we?

right . . . that's the problem. The "we" I mean is the other people who can help you. if it's just I, of course things will be the same. that's the problem.

I can't rely on others! No one can; I should be able to help myself. Right?

if you could do this by yourself, you would. no, no, no. you need to rely on others. you shouldn't be able to do this by yourself. (you can't . . . history shows that.)

???? I know what you mean, but that makes me very, very vulnerable.

yep . . . vulnerable and powerless.

This really sux.

yes it does.

Why can't I just be like any other large person who goes to WW and loses the weight?

I'd have to ask you the same question.

I have no answer. Because I don't have enough willpower? I don't care about myself? I don't care that I can't fit into any clothes???

maybe the answer is simply you need to go along a different path.

powerless path?

many of the paths are powerless paths. WW could be a powerless path. the person says "man, I just can't do this . . . can you guys help me? you tell me what to do and I'll do it!"

I think I can live with that.

you'll need to make yourself vulnerable . . . become open to help.

what happens to me is I get a week or 10 days of proper behavior, and then little by

you've done that before in therapy, or it would not have been helpful.

little start to cheat, then binge, and then disappear . . . and the feeling like a failure kicks right in.

sounds like you need help with relapse prevention.

yes. The black and white thinking really was the key for me back on grey sheet.

you need to figure out how to avoid the cheating, or what triggers the cheating.

Even tho the food plan was stringent, I remember once my brother-in-law made some tomato sauce and asked me to taste it. I had already eaten and said no. He said just a tsp full! And I said sorry, no way. 1 extra bite triggers the cheating, gary. There are days I can handle pasta, in measured amounts, and would lose weight (on WW).

yes ... does your family know how much you struggle with this?

Well, my parents don't mention my weight anymore, ever. My husband and friends sure do, yes.

what was your brother-in-law doing? didn't he know?

He didn't think tomato sauce was a big deal. Then I explained and he backed right off, tho.

good ... the ones closest to you have to understand ... that can be quite helpful to you.

My husband is wonderful, so patient. He wants us to have a baby and my life has been on hold. He'd help me with any food plan I was on.

so there are many rewards if you can do this :o)

yes, yes, yes. I feel so emotional right now; weepy.

and you feel supported and loved by your husband.

oh yes. and I have some great friends who love me, too.

you are blessed.

Thank you; I believe I am.

I think the work behind you has been a lot of "why?" I think the work ahead is a lot of "what?" developing and sticking to a plan of action.

I have to be black and white with the food plan. But that's OK, right?

what do you have to do to stay abstinent? yes . . .

weigh and measure!!

what do you have to do today to prevent a relapse?

Not have that extra ounce.

how do you change your thinking so that you don't blow it if you do relapse? what we tell alcoholics if they pick up a drink is: "stop drinking!" reach out for help. immediately.

Oh I see—don't get into the binge. But once you blow it, it's so easy to say screw it. But that's just the WRONG way to think. I should be thinking "get over it."

and you are saying "screw it" to your future baby and other things.

but when the compulsion takes over . . . you know how it is. there's no logic here.

by yourself, you can't handle it . . . with others, you can. right, that's the problem. it doesn't make sense.

Ok, I feel clearer now.

how is your spiritual life?

Another roadblock for me in program!!

talk about that.

I believe in God, and I believe he helped me those 3 mos. of success in the program, but all of a sudden he stopped helping me. I know that sounds ridiculous, but that's how I feel. I used to go to church and pray for help, for abstinence, and I would still eat. I gave up on him.

that's not him . . . that's you.

but I went to church!!

God can help me stay sober, but he's not going to knock a drink out of my hand . . . that's for me to take care of.

Then how can he help?

there's not a simple answer to this question . . .

I know—enter roadblock. The great debate, I used to call it.

we can work on that in the future.

ok.

because it is vital . . . and an answer can be found . . . for you. you have the worst part out of the way already . . .

admitting powerlessness?

there are those who recover who are atheists . . . makes it harder.

oh

yes, the admitting powerlessness puts you ahead as well. so, what's your sense about our online work? do you think it can help you?

Well, I feel you're in between my therapist and Dr. Smith. Definitely.

Client B was very therapy-literate, and quite easily opened up and looked at her behavior. In this first session, she discussed the issues that brought her into treatment at this time. I asked about suicidality to see if that was a current concern and, if so, one that would rule out chat room work. We also began the process of determining whether my skill set and personality matched up with her needs. We worked out our respective roles in the therapy process. I felt comfortable, given my experience, in working with her on the issues she presented. We discussed my role as falling somewhere between her former therapist and her psychiatrist. She began to look at her need to be at least somewhat vulnerable and to allow others in her life to help her. Her tendency was to protect herself and to try to do everything all by herself so she didn't have to make herself vulnerable.

After the chat room session presented here, Client B committed to weekly sessions. Here is a transcript of the second session:

[Therapist]: *what do you want to be the focus of our time together?*

[Client B]: I'm not sure; I was thinking of re-entering therapy with either my former therapist or Dr. Smith

instead of online?

In addition to us, I meant.

hmmmmm . . .

Good point—I thought you and I would talk only about addiction issues. But that's not necessarily true, is it. I know you're an MSW, just like my therapist.

that's my background and experience . . . but I do work with a number of issues. yes. CSWR

oh. I told [my former therapist] about us. You remember her?

absolutely . . . :o)

She spoke very highly of you; me and her are great friends.

I used to get a big kick out of her.

:-D

if you do decide to go back, it would be good to sign releases so we could communicate.

I really don't know what to do. Are you saying we can talk about more than just "addiction"

yes . . .

issues? Oh sure, I would sign that release. But I know money will be an issue with her/me. As well as Dr. Smith, and time, now that I've moved. Agh!

well, let's start and you can always make a switch later if needed.

ok

so, list the areas you want to address in treatment.

Gee . . . I guess it would have to be to stop my family from abusing me . . . letting go of the hope they'll be nice and decent to me one day.

maybe I should rephrase that . . .

?

what can you address in treatment . . .

ok . . .

we can't work on what your family will do.

my reactions

yes . . .

my judgment of time spent with them. my feelings of guilt

yes

I gotchya now. my acceptance of myself

so, choices you make which put you in uncomfortable situations with them.

My understanding that they were cruel, I was a good person. yes.

uncomfortable feelings related to your interactions with them.

absolutely.

all workable.

I've come a long way, gary. You don't really know that, but I have.

I believe you from our last talk.

yes.

what else do you want to work on?

My food addiction—its relation to my therapy, or does it stand alone?

it's definitely a problem that needs addressing.

yes.

ok ... anything else?

No ... my baby issues are tied up with the weight issue.

right ... that's a positive outcome when you are successful.

yes.

ok ... we've identified the problems—now the goals? food addiction—goal?

Ok ... to love myself enough to not punish myself with food anymore.

ok ... maybe we should do objectives just to keep from getting confused.

what do you mean?

what specific steps need to be taken to get you to the goal? Manage compulsive overeating and not punish self with food. 1. attend WW

Yes.

2. discuss issues weekly with Gary. what else?

ok ... I have to change my thinking. Once I fall off the wagon it takes me days/weeks to get motivated again.

3. Develop written relapse prevention plan.

Oh ... ok. I wrote those down, btw

4. Write down 5 negative thoughts that keep me overeating once I start. 5. Write down 5 positive thoughts that can get me back on track much more quickly.

ok. I like that; I can answer them easily.

(I'm saying these as suggestions ... you might have suggestions that fit a little better.)

I can sure rattle off those 5 neg. thoughts.

let's keep on tx [treatment] planning . . .

ok

next problem . . .

Seeking family approval.

seeking family approval that isn't forthcoming.

right

goal?

To be confident enough to know, without hesitation, they are wrong. and not obsess over it.

how about to identify and meet my needs outside of my family.

Well, honestly I have a lot of needs already met aside from family.

your husband and friends, heh?

Husband, friends, family, career. I feel very happy with my life for the most part.

goal: trust my reactions/feelings/thoughts when I'm with my family.

yes!

(it's always better to frame a goal as a positive.) (you're writing this down?)

Ok, unlike "not to have self-doubt." yes

right . . . to feel confident!

Confident that I am a good person and that they are cruel.

holding family responsible for their behavior.

Muahaha!

mua?

hahahah. That's a big hearty laugh.

:o) oh . . . like ROFL, heh?

Oh yeah! ROFLMAO!

me too!

you gotta sound it out!

oh, I got it . . . ok . . . what problem is left?

anyway, I laugh because my family would never look at their behavior. It's much easier to blame the scapegoat, me.

that is really sad . . . it's impossible for them to grow.

But I guess it's my reaction that counts, not theirs. They're into denial, minimization and ignoring of my feelings.

and it's funny in that they probably think they are right.

absolutely . . . and that I'm a bitch.

[She talks for a few minutes about her use of language and how when she gets upset, she curses. I normalize that behavior. We then start talking about feelings.]

that's the other problem . . . feelings management.

yes.

problems with feelings management. goal—manage feelings.

I tend to obsess over things.

Objectives: 1. identify and express feelings directly. 2. take responsibility for feelings related to family issues. 3. get further grounded in the facts about feelings. (we can do all these things online.)

Ok . . . great. How do you feel about a supplemental visit f2f here and there?

whatever works for you, I'll support.

You do see people f2f?

yes

do you see people privately where you work?

yes, I rent an office there.

Ok.

you are welcome.

Do you think it would be helpful? say, once a month?

do you think it would be helpful?

Yes

we'll do it then.

There are benefits of f2f that you can't capture online.

yes.

I never liked phone sessions with Dr. Smith. Never did them with my therapist. I always felt he was doing something else while talking to me. I don't feel that way online, tho.

hmmm. yeah, we both have to pay attention. so, you have a good sense of what we will be working on? do you agree with the tx plan?

Sure; those are my core issues. It seems like a ton of stuff. You know what really pisses me off . . .

what?

I've been in therapy on and off for about 10 years with my therapist, then Smith. I still have stuff to work on!!! When will this ever, ever end??

I don't know how to answer that question . . . sometimes folks go in and out of tx for awhile.

I can answer the quest . . .

then, they are out of tx. with occasional recharges after that.

I've come a long way. My hx [history] is horrendous; my abuse has been horrific . . . I've come a long, long way, but I guess I have to just accept I'm not done yet.

hmm . . . it's funny how we can answer our own questions :o)

I do it all the time :-)

In this session, I focused on beginning the treatment planning process. Client B had a pretty clear sense of what her issues were and readily identified them, but initially focused on how others had to change. A simple reminder from me to keep the focus on herself through a reframing of the initial question was enough to get her on the right track. It was important for her to identify her issues and to look at ways in which each issue could be addressed. She accepted the objectives I suggested, and would benefit from creating her own as the treatment progressed. She brought up the idea of our work including sessions in person once per month. She also understood that she had made substantial progress in previous treatment.

The next transcript is part of a session Client B and I had in the middle of her treatment:

[Therapist]: so the process has been you get gung ho, someone bursts the bubble and then you give up.

[Client B]: yep. Or I burst the bubble.

hmmm . . . well, that's got to change . . .

Yes—it all comes back to the orig. problem of trusting my own instincts.

and you've been around long enough to know . . . there's not a quick fix to most of our problems . . .

I know this will be a life-long thing for me. No doubt about it.

the lasting change comes from slow, hard work.

Whether I'm on an 1800, 1200 or 2500 cal plan to maintain, I will always need help.

so we have to get excited to do the hard work!

I just remembered something my therapist used to always say: that I do fine on a diet "when I'm in the good, positive mood to." But once the other negative stuff kicks in, I blow it, can't fight it.

right . . . it's the same with all of us . . .

I guess so, but I think of those words and I feel lousy about myself.

it's easy to act like a Christian when everyone's lovey dovey. the true test is when you are around someone nasty.

I know.

it's easy to stay sober when you are in an AA meeting. but we have to stay sober in the real world.

its about when you leave.

right

So according to my therapist, I feel doomed then. or, I am doomed.

well, it's true that you won't always feel up and excited. we just have to have a plan to deal with that.

right, but she always made me feel like she expected me to fail. And believe me, I'm not shy, I told her this.

you've associated uncomfortable feelings with failure.

Doesn't everyone?

no

cannot compute. cannot imagine.

that's a problem.

hmmm. Well, as a kid/teen, whenever I didn't do well in something I was attacked. Verbally and physically; called names, etc. Gee, might that be where this comes from? Never sweetly encouraged that it was OK.

you know it is.

oh yeah

doesn't make it right or doesn't make it the way it was supposed to be. it's part of your relearning.

what do you mean doesn't make it right, etc?

you were mistreated . . . even though your attackers felt justified, or thought they were right, they were not . . . it was not right.

Oh—of course not.

but you have this belief . . . even though it's not right. discomfort = failure. the new learning is: discomfort = discomfort.

I can hear echoing in my head my father's voice: YOU ALWAYS WANT TO TAKE SHORTCUTS!!!! Gary, I've had to relearn just about every basic I was taught.

you need a new message . . . "the simplest is the most profound."

hmmmm

"if it works, it's good"

In my family, we were never encouraged to have our own minds.

if you find a diet today that helps you, and that you feel good about, that's a good thing.

And I'm very thrilled with the TOPS [Take Off Pounds Sensibly] package thus far. And am doing very well.

now, you understand that you have your own mind . . . you are not hooked up by electrodes to other family members . . . you are not a part of a network of brains . . . :o) your mind is your mind.

I do ... and I use it ... but sometimes parts of me get sucked back in, even temporarily.

it is no one else's.

My mother always told me how smart I was, and then when I started to 2nd guess her, she told

so ... back to the point ...

me I was a know-it-all that should come off my "high horse." Ugh!

if you feel uncomfortable because of feedback from another ... you need to manage that discomfort without causing yourself more problems.

Manage it by setting limits.

it's not helpful for you to then say "screw it" ... you are screwing yourself in the deal.

Yes! isn't setting limits on negative people the way to go?

maybe setting limits in your interactions with others, yes.

Yes.

we can't control others ... you can't have your other therapist act in ways that you want.

True, but I can choose to keep distance.

but you can (and have) set limits with others.

Yes.

and hold true to the reality of the moment.

A great old saying of mine: You can't choose your family, but you can choose not to bother with them.

you are absolutely correct.

Will I always have setbacks? As much as I've learned in therapy, sometimes I forget to apply it and I get sucked in. Will I always be prone to this?

I think it will be less so once you get down to a weight you are comfortable with.

Hmmm. I really believe I'm on my way, Gary. This program has the tools to help me. To help myself.

When you are there . . . you will feel much less vulnerable. now . . . when someone says something . . . it touches a tremendous amount of pain in you.

it can. especially if I'm off guard.

and you can eat to deal with that pain . . . when you are closer to your goal . . . you'll be in less pain. and more able to say "well, screw you!!" if that's what needs to be said.

More confident.

yep. more proud, happy, accomplished and so on.

Client B started the session by talking about how she would get upset when her former therapist reminded her of her inability to stick with a diet plan. The work in the moment was to avoid getting caught up in her feelings toward her previous therapist and at the same time to support her in her efforts to begin and to maintain an appropriate plan for managing food. She then talked about family issues and their continuing impact on her.

The work with Client B went on for approximately another month. She seemed comfortable with the eating plan she put in place and developed a support system to help her stay on the right track. We never did meet in person. She asked to stop the therapy because of financial considerations. Upon followup in the fall of 2000, she reported doing well.

Long-Term Chat Room Therapy

Client C saw my profile on AOL and e-mailed me about possible treatment. Her father was an active alcoholic, and she wanted to address issues related to that as well as issues related to her feeling "overwhelmed." We met in a chat room on AOL, and I spent about 90 minutes assessing her.

Client C was in her mid-30s and worked full time outside of the home. She reported having a number of friends. However, she had not been able to reveal her emotional life to anyone, including family members. She felt "overwhelmed" because her inability to open up to others resulted in her having to deal with her feelings by herself although she lacked appropriate skills to do so. She seemed to struggle with common issues of adult children of alcoholics: unresolved shame, lack of self-care skills, difficulty dealing with feelings, and problems in identifying and meeting her own needs. I believed my skill set and experience qualified me to work with her on those issues. I became committed to the process of helping her online when she told me how she had previously sought help from another online "therapist" who in the first session verbally sexually abused her by questioning her in detail about her marital sexual activities when her sexuality was not a part of her presenting problem at all. I recommended that she participate in Al-Anon, but she refused. She said she could not share her problems with others in person. She reported that she had been to a psychiatrist on several occasions, but was so uncomfortable because of his aloofness and coldness that she refused to go back. She also refused to consider any other therapy in person.

The following transcript illustrates the quality of interaction possible in long-term chat room therapy:

[Therapist]: what do you want to focus on tonight?

[Client C]: I don't know . . . I feel kind of blah

physically or emotionally?

emotionally I think

ok. can you talk about what the feeling(s) are?

well I guess I'm just tired of thinking about everything . . . does that make sense?

is it tired of thinking or tired of feeling?

I don't know

ok. Why don't you continue the thought that you started above . . . I guess I'm just tired of . . . ok?

lol! you know . . . I just wish I could either say . . . "Do over" and start all over again . . . or

or what?

<sigh> or take "my stuff" and bundle it up and put it in a box and choose something else and start over . . . :o)

ok. I wonder what you could do that would be close to either one of those choices?

nothing . . . I'm stuck with what I got . . . there are no "do overs" in life

are there any "I live with what I've got, but do the rest differently?"

sure . . . but no matter what . . . there is always that . . . "what I've got"

what do you mean? what do you have?

well . . . not just what I have . . . but I mean . . . I can't change anything that has happened up until 1 second ago . . . everything I did 20 years ago . . . anything I said this morning . . .

yes

what I just said to you 3 minutes ago . . . I can't change

right

and no matter what . . . you can't escape it

right

I can't leave tonight . . . and go to Hawaii . . . and get away from everything or anything

(even if you went to Hawaii, you couldn't get away, right?)

the last couple of days . . . I've been thinking of some things my grandmother used to say to me. 1. If you want sympathy . . . look it up in the dictionary . . . and 2. you need broad shoulders and a big brain to handle everything that comes along because you have to take care of everything yourself . . . no one is going to help you

did she live in tough times?

I guess so . . . Chicago, early 1900s

do you believe what she said? has that been your experience?

yeah . . . I think she was right

has that been your experience?

yes

why are you bringing this up when you talk about wanting to get away?

I don't know

it might be that there is much wisdom in what she said, but there is more.

more of what?

It just doesn't go far enough. It's good to have broad shoulders and a big brain. and it's good to take care of things yourself. and there are many good people out there who can help you if you allow it to happen. People don't need sympathy and whining is very unattractive ;o)

lol

but empathy is a different thing. Empathy (the ability to feel with another) is part of the human condition and wonderful when it happens between people. and is much different from sympathy or pity. It helps the receiver feel "a part of" and "not alone." does this make sense?

yes

you've not let people help you in the past. and I haven't seen you, but I imagine your shoulders to be broad. and you seem to have a good brain.

lol

you've listened to what she has said. now you're hearing the rest of it. not to conflict, but to complement.

I don't understand

you don't need to look for sympathy from others . . .

I don't want sympathy from anyone . . .

that's ok. the learning is about empathy . . . opening up to others. as you choose. I guess I'm having trouble explaining myself.

not really . . . I understand

do you see me as helping you at times?

oh definitely . . . :o)

so what she said may be true much of the time, but not all of the time. you don't have to figure this out all by yourself.

:o)

you're opening up to me and this process is helping me help you. do you see your openness as a big change for you?

oh yeah . . . sometimes I still can't believe it. lol

yea . . . pretty cool!

:o)

ok . . . what I'm trying to say is if you live by the philosophy that no one will help you, and you don't allow others to help you, no one can help you, even if they want to. your openness allows that to change. good for you.

lol

Client C shared a family motto that had effectively precluded her ability to reach out or to open up to others. The work in the session was to honor the family motto while extending it to allow her to share some of her burdens with others. I used our relationship and her developing openness to illustrate the need to be open to others and the appropriateness of that openness. She made very good progress and developed more awareness of the defenses that had kept others out of her life.

Client C went on to therapy in person, which was prompted by her revealing an eating disorder that was more appropriately treated in person. Chat room therapy was stopped after she agreed to seek and was able to engage with a therapist in person. Her ability to engage in therapy in person reflected the degree of change that had been facilitated, at least in part, by chat room therapy. She had also been able to develop several relationships with peers and was able to talk about her feelings and issues with them and to get support from them.

Conclusions

Therapy in a chat room can be conducted in an ethical and skillful manner with clients who are appropriate for this level of care. The chat room therapist, in addition to being skilled in face-to-face therapy, must have a skill set that allows him or her to interact comfortably and effectively online. Just as not all clients are appropriate for chat room therapy, not all therapists can appropriately provide it.

As the number of therapists who use this medium grows, research will be needed to verify the efficacy of therapy in a chat room. Specific interventions and their effectiveness also need to be explored. Training and supervision of online therapists is an emerging area that will be quite important in the next several years. Supervision is possible online as well (Stofle & Hamilton, 1998).

Kottler (1991) reports that there are "certain moments or events in therapy that would be considered significant by almost all practitioners" (p. 44). These events signify progress in therapy. Kottler (1991, pp. 45–46) listed six events from Mahrer and Nadler:

1. Revealing significant material about self.
2. Sharing personal and meaningful feelings.
3. Exploring issues that have previously been warded off.
4. Demonstrating a degree of insight into the meaning and implications of behavior.
5. Being highly expressive and vibrant in communications.
6. Sharing strong positive feelings toward the therapist and the way things are progressing.

The transcripts in this chapter illustrate that some of these moments are possible when utilizing only text-based chat. The sense of presence (Lombard & Ditton, 1997), along with the disinhibition associated with communicating through a computer, allow significant information to be disclosed more rapidly. If the therapist is skilled in online interaction, he or she can use the client's openness to facilitate change more rapidly. The depth of the client's sharing and the skill of the therapist enhance the therapeutic relationship. That paves the way for client growth and change, at heart the purpose of therapy.

References

Ainsworth, M. (n.d.). *Confidentiality: Is it safe to talk?* [Online]. Available: www.metanoia. org/imhs/safety.htm

Barak, A. (1999). Psychological applications on the Internet: A discipline on the threshold of a new millennium. *Applied and Preventive Psychology, 8,* 231–246.

Childress, C. (1998). *Potential risks and benefits of online psychotherapeutic interventions* [Online]. Available: www.ismho.org/issues/9801.htm

Fink, J. (1999). *How to use computers and cyberspace in the clinical practice of psychotherapy.* Northvale, NJ: Jason Aronson.

Grohol, J. (1997). *Why online psychotherapy? Because there is a need* [Online]. Available: psychcentral.com/archives/n102297.htm

Grohol, J. (1999). *Best practices in e-therapy: Confidentiality and privacy* [Online]. Available: psychcentral.com/best/best2.html

Gross, S. J. (2000). *Internet characteristics and the ethical issues raised by online counseling* [Online]. Available: www.helphorizons.com/vo/library/articles.asp?id=89

Hartwell-Walker, M. (2000). *Coming soon: Web therapy* [Online]. Available: www. helphorizons.com/vo/library/article.asp?id=123

Holmes, L. (n.d.). *Why this is not therapy* [Online]. Available: netpsych.com/share/nottx.htm

Holmes, L. (1997). *You can't do psychotherapy on the Net, yet* [Online]. Available: mentalhealth.about.com/health/mentalhealth/library/weekly/aa010499.htm

International Society of Mental Health Online & Psychiatric Society for Informatics. (2000). *Suggested principles for the online provision of mental health services* [Online]. Available: www.ismho.org/suggestions.html

Kottler, J. A. (1991). *The compleat therapist.* San Francisco: Jossey-Bass.

Lombard, M., & Ditton, T. (1997). At the heart of it all: The concept of presence. *Journal of Computer Mediated Communication* [Online], *3*(2). Available: www.ascusc.org/jcmc/vol3/issue2/lombard.html

Maheu, M. (1999). *Telehealth: Re-tooling psychology for the 21st century* [Online]. Available: telehealth.net/articles/article2.html

Ohio Department of Rehabilitation and Correction, Adult Parole Authority. (n.d.). *Older offender training instructor manual.* Columbus: Author.

Sanderson, W. C., & Woody, S. (Eds.). (1995). *Manuals for empirically validated treatments* [Online]. Available: psychcentral.com/txmanul.htm

Seligman, M. E. P. (1995). The effectiveness of psychotherapy: The Consumer Reports Study. *American Psychologist* [Online], *50,* 965–974. Available: www.apa.org/journals/seligman.html

Shulman, R. (2000). Lost confidence and confidentiality in psychotherapy. *Perspectives* [Online], *5*(4). Available: mentalhelp.net/perspectives/articles/art09620003.htm

Stofle, G. (1997). *Thoughts about online psychotherapy: Ethical and practical implications* [Online]. Available: members.aol.com/stofle/onlinepsych.htm

Stofle, G. (2001). *Choosing an online therapist: A step-by-step guide to finding professional help on the Web.* Harrisburg, PA: White Hat Communications.

Stofle, G., & Hamilton, S. (1998). Online supervision. *The New Social Worker* [Online], 5(4). Available: www.socialworker.com/onlinesu.htm

Suler, J. (2000). *Psychotherapy in cyberspace* [Online]. Available: www.rider/edu/users/suler/psycyber/therapy/html

Suler, J., & Fenichel, M. (2000). *The Online Clinical Case Study Group of the International Society of Mental Health Online: A report from the Millennium Group* [Online]. Available: www.rider.edu/users/suler/psycyber/casegrp.html

Wylie, M. (2000). *Mental health therapy online holds promise, dangers* [Online]. Available: www.newhouse.com/archive/story1a.html

6

Clinical Principles
to Guide the Practice
of E-Therapy

Peter M. Yellowlees

MANY THERAPISTS already practice on the Internet. However, it is fascinating that a proportion of them seem to have forgotten the basic principles that guide good clinical practice. They seem to treat e-therapy as if it were some new process of treatment, some new form of clinical care. Some are prepared to treat patients who remain anonymous. Others deny they are giving mental health treatment at all, preferring to call it advice or information, yet they still charge for it. On the Internet, practitioners from a variety of professional backgrounds propose to answer specific questions from consumers at a rate of a dollar per question, as if they were sitting in a booth at a fair. What these practitioners forget is that the type of e-therapy that will survive and flourish will surely be underpinned by the same basic principles as is good in-person practice.

After all, e-therapy is simply an extension of therapy in person. The basic clinical principles are the same, although with some extensions and additions that take into account the virtual relationship. The two approaches may well be integrated into a package of care that incorporates both. In particular, it is important for e-therapists to be flexible, respectful, competent, and responsible. In the future, clinical accountability and the promotion of self-care by patients will be increasingly emphasized.

The Internet in Real-World Practice

Tom Ferguson (1998) advocated using the Internet as a routine extension of "real-world" practice to add extra services, provide more information, and increase access to care. He covered succinctly the sorts of issues that physicians need to consider:

> *Physicians may find it far easier than they think to offer their patients their own personalized blend of highly accessible, high-quality online health resources. In addition to welcoming patient e-mail under appropriate circumstances, physicians might establish their own Web pages with lists of frequently asked patient questions and answers and annotated links to useful and authoritative medical Web sites. Physicians could also provide biographical information, explain their practice philosophy, offer online appointment scheduling, and point to high-quality health databases and directories of online support groups.*
>
> *Such resources could serve current patients, help attract new ones, and might even allow physicians to budget their own time more effectively. Clinicians who invite their patients to join them in electronic conversation may reap another benefit as well—a better appreciation for the "other" side of their patient/physician relationship, which has commanded increased attention and has come under increased pressure in recent years. (p. 1362)*

In today's increasingly competitive world, mental health practitioners who do not have an Internet presence, are not prepared to use e-mail, and are not able to deal with Internet-savvy patients are likely to be significantly disadvantaged. The first step, then, is to incorporate the Internet into "normal," real-world care.

Basic Clinical Principles

Let us now look in more detail at the basic clinical principles that guide good e-therapy practice.

Be Flexible

Although mental health practitioners always need to adapt their techniques to individual patients in order to ensure appropriate treatment, these practitioners must be even more flexible once they begin treating patients online. Although practitioners cannot afford to spend several hours a day looking up the latest findings on every psychiatric disorder, patients are motivated to research their problems, and family members of patients may use online resources to an even greater extent. Clinicians must get used to being confronted with large amounts of information—much of it unreliable, but much of it excellent—and be flexible enough to analyze, review critically, and critique this information with patients. To employ these skills, however, practitioners must be open to the changed nature of the therapist-patient relationship and understand that patient-driven care is not only here to stay, but will continue to spread.

Mental health professionals must be able to integrate information about mental illness from a wide variety of sources and cultural contexts. For example, in Western medicine we talk about evidence-based practice. We spend a lot of time attempting to provide best-evidence mental health care and to ensure that our normal, day-to-day practice is underpinned by reliable research results, ideally from double-blind, randomized, controlled trials. Practitioners of Eastern medicine, however, may take the view that their practice is underpinned by 2,000 or more years of experience, which is enough evidence for them. As the Web opens up the world to us, we have to be flexible enough to cross cultural and societal boundaries.

Clinicians also have to live their lives flexibly. The world no longer follows a 5-day workweek. The world is, to use jargon, "24/7." Businesspeople operate continuously. Global corporations frequently have teams in different time zones take turns so that the work never stops and projects are completed twice as rapidly. Practitioners now have to realize that they are part of the business world. Increasingly, we will need to take an enterprise approach to mental health care and collaborate with different groups and businesses at different times. We can no longer think of ourselves as being the center or key player in the health care environment. We must have the flexibility to work in teams, collaborate with health professionals of other disciplines, and work with people who have nonclinical areas of expertise; particularly, in the virtual world, with experts in information technology and information management.

Be Respectful

On the Internet, it does not matter who you are, what disabilities you have, or what your background is. The Internet is one of the most egalitarian environments ever created; it has given patients a new voice. Patients now have the opportunity to define what specific treatments they wish to receive and what in general they believe qualifies as good mental health care. For example, the best advice for psychiatrists that I have read was posted by Louise Sullivan (1998), writing on her own experience of depression. Her suggestions, which I have summarized, were:

1. Treat the patient with the utmost dignity and respect.
2. Assume that explanations of the illness are required.
3. Listen to and see the patient regularly, especially early in treatment.
4. Explain and monitor medications and symptoms.
5. Insist on hospitalization if it is indicated.
6. Be encouraging and hopeful.
7. Only use psychotherapy when the patient has recovered from the initial symptoms of depression and is well enough for it.
8. Remain available until the patient has fully recovered.

Note that Sullivan focused on the issues of dignity and respect first. The change in the balance of power between patients and practitioners means that respect, in its widest definition, is increasingly important.

The ubiquitous availability of information on the Internet (Yellowlees, 2000) surely helps to break down the destructive stigma and secrecy surrounding mental illness and to make it more socially acceptable to receive treatment. Giving patients the respect they are due also helps.

Therapists have to acknowledge the fundamental rights, dignity, and worth of their patients. For example, just as therapists may wish to have a degree of privacy and not be bombarded by e-mails from patients, so do patients have the same rights, and therapists have to make sure that their patients don't mind being e-mailed themselves. Imagine the difficulties that might occur if therapists e-mailed patients at their work e-mail addresses, and this led to employers learning intimate details about the patients' personal lives. In addition to privacy and confidentiality, therapists have to understand issues of self-determination and autonomy in the virtual world.

Be Competent

Unfortunately, a proportion of mental health practitioners are clinically incompetent, either through a lack of training or continuing education, or because they have become unwell in some way. Practitioners in the real world have been less than perfect at self-regulation, and it is still relatively uncommon for clinicians to be deregistered or barred in some other way from practicing their profession. Professional associations have many concerns about the practice of e-therapy, from whether charlatans will use it to make a quick buck to whether it will be as effective as in-person care. Medical practitioners in many countries now have to undergo continuing education and recertification in order to keep their professional qualifications. This is not yet the case for all mental health professionals, but it should be.

A variety of principles of good clinical practice have been proposed. The American Medical Informatics Association (Kane & Sands, 1998) published guidelines, intended for doctors but also relevant to other therapists, on the use of e-mail for clinical and administrative purposes. Their recommendations, which I have summarized, include:

- Don't use e-mail for urgent matters, because you cannot be sure when e-mail will be answered—use the phone or communicate in person.
- Ensure that your patients know how to reach you by e-mail, how and where you store e-mail, and whether you copy it and place it in your medical records.
- Decide with your patients for what general purposes they may communicate with you using e-mail and have them specify the general purpose of each e-mail in its subject line so that you can deal with it quickly. Where possible, use terms known only to your patients.
- Ensure that your patients know they can phone you or your office if they do not get an e-mail response within an agreed period of time, say, 48 hours.
- Don't forward possibly identifying material about your patients to third parties without your patients' expressed consent.
- Encrypt e-mail if possible. This may not be practical because both parties have to have and to know how to use compatible encryption software. If encryption is not possible, ensure that your patients understand that e-mail is not secure.

Other useful guidelines have been produced by the American Telemedicine Association (ATA, 1999) and the National Board for Certified Counselors (NBCC, 1997). A comprehensive discussion of such guidelines is included in "Your Guide to E-Health" (Yellowlees, 2001).

Apart from following various guidelines to ensure competent practice, therapists have to recognize the limitations of their expertise and provide only the services and apply only the techniques for which they are properly qualified. Therapists who are poor at writing or typing should probably avoid using e-mail in their practices. Therapists have to be fair, honest, and aware of their limitations. The claims made by some e-therapists are quite ridiculous. Beware the Internet "colleague" who offers to cure patients rapidly of a wide variety of diseases. The reality of mental health treatment is that if it takes significant time and energy in person, it is probably going to be even more difficult online, although in-person and online approaches may be complementary.

In order to practice competently online, a health professional must possess good computer skills. Despite the fact that computer technology is becoming more user-friendly and e-mail in particular is already extremely simple to use, many therapists are still technologically incompetent. Many are afraid to learn. In the same way that radiologists must be able to use imaging equipment to take X-rays, psychiatrists working online must have a working knowledge of computers. They need to have the skills to work in virtual environments and to involve a variety of other health professionals and patients' families. They should also be proficient in searching the Internet so that they can provide good-quality information for their patients. They should be administratively competent: Their online booking and billing procedures must be efficient; their records, whether electronic or paper-based, must be properly maintained; and their procedures must be organized, clearly explained, and easy to understand.

Finally, online practitioners as well as face-to-face therapists must be able to analyze their treatment outcomes and to compare them with those of colleagues and those in the literature. Research skills are particularly important for e-therapists, given the paucity of available information about e-therapy. Mental health practitioners who have significant virtual practices should continually review their methods and publish, either in academic journals or on the Web, the results of their endeavors so that others may learn from them. Currently there is little evidence to support the use of the Internet in mental health care, particularly for consultations, and building this evidence base is of crucial importance to our finding out not only what works, but what works best, with whom, and how.

Be Responsible

Therapists have to uphold the same standards of ethical and professional conduct in the virtual world as they do in the real world. Perhaps the single most important action that e-therapists can encourage is for patients to seek second opinions if they wish. Responsible therapists do not get upset when their patients ask for second opinions, because they and their patients have nothing to fear and everything to gain.

Responsible, accountable clinical practice is especially necessary on the Internet; one of the advantages for patients in the virtual world is that they often retain a perfect copy of any advice or consultations that they receive. That may give them good ammunition if they ever have concerns about their practitioners or complain to health professional regulatory boards. There cannot be much argument with signed e-mails from therapists to patients, whereas there are frequently major difficulties when the "evidence" is simply perceptions or recollections of what went on in person.

Potential Online Problems

There are several potential problems in the world of virtual mental health of which patients and therapists need to be aware. These include not only Internet addiction and "cyberchondria," but also the possibility of deceptive marketing, poor advice, and dishonest relationships (Yellowlees, 2000).

Internet addiction is becoming increasingly recognized, yet we know little about those who become so addicted. Some people spend many hours each day on the Internet, often surfing aimlessly or developing a whole world of virtual relationships that are based on fantasy rather than reality. Such people frequently use the Internet to avoid difficulties in their life or as a substitute for friendship, love, or other interests. Marriages and families may suffer. Doctors seem particularly prone to this syndrome. Many doctors are, by the nature of their training, rather obsessional and dependent. Both personality traits are helpful in the real world, but may lead to problems in the virtual world. Such doctors may start to spend too much time trying to find the latest information to help their patients or too much energy trying to develop the perfect Web site for their practice. The Internet is, despite everything that is said about it, still a false or virtual world, and although we can have relationships over it, work in it, and use it, it is not a replacement for the real world and never will be. Doctors need to recognize this syndrome, to understand that they are perhaps more likely than the average person to be afflicted by it, and to make sure that they do not encourage it in their patients.

Some patients who, in the real world, might have had hypochondria, now—with access to the Internet—have cyberchondria. They misinterpret physical or psychological symptoms and spend hours surfing Web sites trying to find information about causes and treatments. These are the patients who in the past came to consultations with medical dictionaries or pharmaceutical books, usually followed by copious handwritten notes including pages describing their symptoms. The immediacy and accessibility of the Internet has meant that some of these patients have been able to move online with their hypochondria. The large amount of information—both true and false—on the Internet fuels their concerns and makes them more anxious and worried. I have already seen several patients like this. The only treatment that I could really offer them was "withdrawal" from Internet. In one instance, this meant asking a student to move out of his student lodgings and return home to his parents, who did not have an Internet connection. This intervention finally prevented him from sitting up all night trying to find the latest and greatest biological "cure" for his symptoms.

Other problems on the Web of which clinicians need to be aware and warn patients about include:

- *Deceptive marketing:* Many Web sites that purport to be health sites only use a health focus to draw people into them.
- *Poor or biased advice:* Patients are increasingly participating in anonymous meetings in chat rooms or getting pulled into quasi-scientific or religious cults that have very different motives for their existence than the provision of virtual health care. It can sometimes be extremely difficult to identify which organizations or groups are actually behind such Web sites. Clinicians need to discuss this issue openly with their patients, so that the patients can learn to critically evaluate sites for reliability and validity (Yellowlees, 2000).
- *Dishonest relationships:* There are men who cross-dress virtually, pretending on the Internet to be women. They start up relationships posing as women and continue, sometimes for months, to deceive others who may develop very strong feelings of affection or even love for them (Yellowlees, 2001). There have also been several cases of people being "stalked" on the Web; one man was jailed recently for having advertised on the Internet his ex-girlfriend as someone who might provide sadomasochistic sexual services. He even supplied the woman's address.

Clinicians who work in the virtual world have to understand its downsides and possible resultant complications. The issues just discussed have become evident after only a few years of mass Internet use, and there will doubtless be additional problems in the future. It makes clinical sense for these risks to be discussed openly with patients who frequent the Internet or are being treated online, to ensure that they do not become unwitting victims of or suffer further difficulties from the virtual world or the people who inhabit it.

An Example of Good E-Therapy Practice

An example of good e-therapy practice is that provided by Doctor Global (www.doctorglobal.com), where I hold the position of Executive Director of the Mental Health Program. At Doctor Global, patients are treated only by registered clinicians. Once patients register and provide basic demographic details, they are able to choose their clinicians much as they would in person, based on the biographies and photographs published on the Web site. In the case of the Mental Health Clinic, the clinicians are either psychiatrists or psychologists. The patients complete some straightforward structured interviews and screening tests and respond to very specific questions relevant to their problems. If the results indicate that the patients are seriously depressed or acutely unwell, instant messages are automatically sent urging them to see their primary care providers immediately and telling them not to wait for the Doctor Global clinicians to reply.

For patients deemed not to be seriously depressed or acutely unwell, the next step is that their consultations are directed to the relevant Doctor Global clinicians, who guarantee to reply to the patients within 48 hours. These replies are reasonably detailed and usually include probable differential diagnoses and management advice. If the patients wish additional input, they can of course immediately consult further with the clinicians who already are familiar with the patients' information.

The patients may review their evaluations. One of the obvious advantages of this approach is that the patients may also use their Doctor Global assessments as "second opinions," printing them out and discussing them with local practioners.

All clinicians working for Doctor Global undergo quality audits of both their clinical and their written communication skills. Also, a proportion of their consultations are reviewed by the Clinical Advisory Committee (of which I am a member). These evaluations ensure that the clinical advice the clinicians give and the e-mail communication approaches they take are of high quality. As part of the training and accreditation process, clinicians working for Doctor Global have all their professional registration papers checked and must perform a minimum of five trial consultations that are reviewed by the Clinical Advisory Committee. The following is an explanation of this process:

> Doctor Global consultants follow current "best practice" guidelines. These are based on the highest ethical standards of medical practice and have been adapted and developed where necessary for e-health by the Clinic Directors and the Continuing Medical Education and Quality Assurance Committees of Doctor Global. An editorial board of independent community and professional members assists with the development of practice standards and ethics. In addition Doctor Global and its consultants follow the guidelines promulgated by professional bodies of which they are members. The fundamental principles on which all guidelines are based are for consultants to promote the health and well being of patients and to practice the science and art of medicine to the best of their ability and within the limits of their expertise.
>
> Any complaints regarding our service will be directed to our Quality Assurance Committee and replied to within 7 days. If a dispute is not settled to the satisfaction of both parties, the matter will be referred to an independent medical arbitrator or the Board of Registration of

the medical practitioner involved. Doctor Global consultants consider the interests and well being of our patients as their prime responsibility, exercise the highest ethical standards in all their dealings and activities, commit to an environment of continual improvement and are sensitive and responsive to the needs and values of the communities and countries in which they work. (www.doctorglobal.com/shared/about/codecon.html)

Doctor Global adheres to the Health on the Net (HON) Code of Conduct for Medical and Health Web Sites (1997), and also makes its own code of conduct and ethical guidelines available for patients to read. The comprehensive quality improvement process—incorporating the Clinical Advisory Committee—means that consultations by clinicians at Doctor Global are almost certainly more frequently and carefully reviewed than would be the case if they were working with patients in person. Particularly if the practitioners were in private practice by themselves, their clinical work would almost never be externally audited.

I use Doctor Global as an example of a provider of high-quality e-therapy that is, in essence, simply an extension of and improvement on care provided using sensible clinical principles in the real world. Patients know whom they are consulting, have access to their own records, and receive well-documented feedback in a clinically sound and ethically appropriate manner. Their practitioners are subject to a quality improvement process and, on top of this, Doctor Global also regularly e-mails patients to assess their satisfaction with their consultations, as well as to get other feedback.

E-Therapy of the Future

The issue of clinical accountability is the defining practice issue that will, I believe, result in the success or failure of e-therapy. If clinicians are not fully accountable for their mistakes, the Internet will become a clinical wasteland ruled by fear. It is for this reason that quality improvement practices such as those introduced by Doctor Global are essential, and that clinicians must have access to audits of their work.

In the Internet environment, it seems inevitable that consumers' health records will be held electronically and that consumers will have access to and control over them. This is standard practice at Doctor Global, and was recently recommended for all of Australia by the National Electronic Health Records Taskforce (2000). Consequently, Australia is moving to develop a national electronic health information network, called HealthConnect, that will allow consumers to control their electronic health records. Logically, it would

FIGURE 6.1
FROM INDUSTRIAL AGE MEDICINE TO
INFORMATION AGE HEALTH CARE

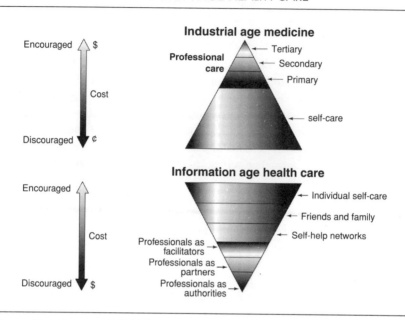

Source: From Ferguson, T. (1995). Consumer Health Infomatics. *Healthcare Forum Journal* *38*(1): 28–33. Adapted with permission of the author.

eventually be possible for these records to be accessed and contributed to by both patients and clinicians during the course of e-therapy.

There will be increasing use of electronic screening tests before consultations, as in the Mental Health Clinic at Doctor Global. Also, the advent of the ubiquitous availability of information systems around the world will promote self-care by patients. Thomas Ferguson (1995) recently described the radical shift—from the industrial age medicine of the past to the information age health care of the future—in the way health services are delivered (see Figure 6.1).

Ferguson described how most of the costs of industrial age medicine were taken up by the professional sectors, with relatively little importance placed on self-care. He asserted that in information age health care the majority of costs would be focused on the three levels of self-care: individual self-care, care from friends and family, and self-help networks. He then saw three different roles for health professionals: as facilitators, as partners, and, to a lesser extent, as authorities.

If we take Ferguson's model and apply it to e-therapy, the results are fascinating. At the first level, individual self-care, the following are important:

- Access to timely, accurate information.
- Conventional and complementary information, including the latest news and updates as well as professional-level information from databases such as Medline (www.nlm.nih.gov) and PsycInfo (www.apa.org/psycinfo).
- The ability to find best-practice and evidence-based personalized treatment guidelines that have no commercial bias.
- Access to information about individual therapists' strengths, skills, and treatment outcomes.
- The creation of personal longitudinal health records, including accounts of past illnesses and treatments.

All of these important therapeutic options are increasingly becoming available. The next level of self-care, care from friends and family, incorporates:

- Access to timely, accurate information—both conventional and complementary—from a caregiver perspective.
- The ability to find best-practice and evidence-based personalized treatment guidelines that have no commercial bias and that include advice for family members.
- Access to information about individual therapists' strengths, skills, and treatment outcomes, as well as about caregiver support groups and networks.

The third level of self-care, self-help networks, includes:

- The provision of "mates" or "guides" for specific Web sites or for specific topics—for example, Leonard Holmes, a psychologist at About (www.about.com), has set up a group of these guides (often consumers themselves) to assist others in finding appropriate information from a particular site or set of links.
- Access to chat rooms, discussion lists, and relevant "experts" for interactive advice.
- Access to second opinions from other consumers and therapists about particular therapists, schools of thought, support groups, and so on.
- The primary prevention of mental health problems in settings such as schools.

Once a patient has made the decision to approach a therapist, both of them need to understand the different types of roles that the therapist might take. Ferguson's first defined role is therapist as *facilitator*. Here the therapist guides the consumer to appropriate information to allow the consumer to make informed treatment choices. The therapist also assists the consumer in accessing appropriate health care, and provides advocacy and perhaps referrals elsewhere.

At the second level, with the therapist as *partner*, the relationship may well involve joint research into therapeutic options. The consumer, who usually has more time and immediate motivation, may be the researcher, whereas the therapist may assist with direction and information analysis. Following a biopyschosocial assessment, treatment is provided along conventional lines, but with a strong consumer and team (if others in addition to the patient and the therapist are involved) focus, and with a significant emphasis on the provision of appropriate education and psychological information.

The final role defined by Ferguson is therapist as *authority*. This is the traditional role of the doctor in the doctor-patient relationship. An authoritarian style of relationship will be less common in the future, but will still be necessary when rapid decisions are needed, when acute or inpatient care is required, and in certain legal situations. It will also be adopted when consumers prefer to be told what to do and not to have to make choices or decisions themselves; for example, if they are depressed at the time.

If we put all of this together, what will be the e-therapy of the future? Consumers will increasingly consult on the Internet with experts, support groups, and their own local practitioners, probably using resources such as:

- Specific information that is in multiple forms, such as text and video, and is personalized for people of all ages.
- Improved online diagnostic scales, rating instruments, and screening tests.
- Support groups, chat rooms, and discussion areas, both facilitated and unfacilitated.
- Products and services, from medications to self-help manuals, other books, CDs, and holiday packages; many—especially the written materials—personalized for individual patients.
- Expert professionals and consumer "guides" who interact by e-mail or videoconferencing for straightforward questions or detailed second opinions on a one-off or continuing basis.

This is the exciting part of e-therapy: It broadens the opportunities for us as practitioners to help consumers and to greatly improve the standard of mental health care in general.

Summary

E-therapy is booming. Without any doubt, the key message for both clinicians and patients involved in such treatment is that the provision of Internet-mediated mental health care should be an extension of best-practice care in person. All of the clinical principles underlying care in person are relevant on the Internet. The beauty of the Internet, however, is that it offers not only therapeutic options that are not available in person but also more accountability of the therapist's practice. There is little doubt that within a few years—especially when videomail and videoconferencing become available in broadband Internet environments—e-therapy will be a common, mainstream mental health practice, and patients whose clinicians do not offer these therapeutic options will be considered to be significantly disadvantaged in treatment. As we continuously improve, over time, how we use this new therapeutic tool, both access to care and therapeutic outcomes will benefit.

References

American Telemedicine Association. (1999). *ATA adopts telehomecare clinical guidelines* [Online]. Available: www.atmeda.org/news/list.html

Ferguson, T. (1998). Digital doctoring: Opportunities and challenges in electronic patient–physician communication. *Journal of the American Medical Association, 280*(15), 1361–1362.

Ferguson, T. (1995). Consumer health infomatics. *Healthcare Forum Journal 38* (1): 28–33.

Health on the Net Foundation. (1997). *Health on the Net code of conduct (HONcode) for medical and health websites* [Online]. Available: www.hon.ch/HONcode/Conduct.html

Kane, B., & Sands, D. Z. (1998). Guidelines for the clinical use of electronic mail with patients. *Journal of the American Medical Informatics Association, 5*(1), 104–111.

National Board for Certified Counselors. (1999). *Standards for the ethical practice of webcounseling* [Online]. Available: www.nbcc.org/ethics/wcstandards.htm

National Electronic Health Records Taskforce. (2000). *A health information network for Australia. Canberra, Australia: Commonwealth of Australia Department of Health and Aged Care* [Online]. Available: www.health.gov.au/healthonline/ehr_rep.htm

Smith, R. (1997). The future of healthcare systems. *British Medical Journal, 314*(7093), 1495–1496.

Sullivan, L. (1998, February). *Psychiatrists: How to help the depressed* [Online]. Available: www.mentalhealth.com/story/p52-dps3.html

Yellowlees, P. M. (2000). Healthcare on the Internet: Buyer beware. *Medical Journal of Australia, 173*(11–12), 629–630.

Yellowlees, P. M. (2001). *Your guide to e-health: Third millennium medicine on the Internet.* Brisbane, Australia: University of Queensland Press. [Online.] Available: www.uqp.uq.edu.au/ebooks.html

7

Suggested Principles of Professional Ethics for E-Therapy[1]

Robert C Hsiung

One Scenario

THERAPIST A RECEIVES his Illinois license, rents an office, and opens for business. His practice, however, is slow to grow. He decides to diversify into e-therapy. He creates a Web page as a virtual shingle: "Online Therapy Services, Inc. Get help by secure real-time chat. E-mail now for more information." Patient A, at work in California and taking advantage of the fast Internet connection in his office, sees the page and sends an e-mail: "I'm having an affair with my boss's wife. It's starting to get complicated! Can you help me?" He searches for other e-therapists and starts corresponding with them, too.

Therapist A replies and says he charges $100/hour. Patient A accepts, but reluctantly, because he considers that steep. They start having chat meetings, and Patient A tells Therapist A about his passionate feelings for his boss's wife. The patient and the therapist focus on Patient A's dissatisfaction in his marriage. To fill Therapist A in on the history of the affair, Patient A e-mails him the last 3 years of entries from his electronic diary. Therapist A spends 2 hours reviewing and commenting on the diary entries and enters that time into his automatic billing software.

Therapist A is then unexpectedly called away because of an illness in his family. That same day, the boss's wife calls Patient A at home and gives him an ultimatum: If he doesn't leave his wife, she'll end their affair.

---

[1] This chapter is an update and expansion of a previous report (Hsiung, 2001).

Patient A immediately sends Therapist A an e-mail asking him what he should do. Therapist A uses a regional Internet service provider, however, and doesn't have access where he is staying. Not getting a response, Patient A calls the state licensing board and asks for the phone number for Online Therapy Services, Inc. They have no such entity in their database. Confused and angry, Patient A signs on to a number of self-help message boards and posts warnings to others about Online Therapy Services. Increasingly desperate, he takes, in an attempt to calm himself, a handful of lithium he was prescribed in the past. Meanwhile, the boss, a possessive type, has the company e-mail server searched, as he does each week, for his wife's name and the words *wife, love, sex,* and *affair.* At the same time, because it's the end of the month, Therapist A's billing software automatically sends Patient A an e-mail bill for the month's chat sessions—plus $200, which Patient A is not expecting, for dealing with the diary entries.

Patient A's wife sits down at their home computer to check her e-mail and finds her husband's message to Therapist A about the boss's wife. The Medical Board of California initiates an investigation, determines that Therapist A has violated the California Business and Professions Code, and notifies the Illinois Department of Professional Regulation. Patient A's multiple message board postings are indexed by the major search engines and become the top responses to searches for "Online Therapy Services, Inc." Having taken too much lithium at once, Patient A gets dizzy, falls down some stairs, and breaks his leg. The boss is informed of Patient A's initial e-mail to Therapist A about the boss's wife and fires Patient A.

Opportunity and Danger

Mental health professionals have discovered the new world of the Internet. Exploring it presents not only new opportunities, but also new dangers. Although hypothetical and improbable as a whole, each step of the above scenario is plausible. The clinical and legal principles that will guide the practice of e-therapy will emerge as experience is gained, research is conducted, and legislation is passed. Ethical principles are also needed in this uncharted territory. A map of the ethical hazards will not only protect the pioneers themselves (both patients and therapists), but also reassure the public (both lay and professional) that this new route is safe.

The basic values of professional ethics are beneficence, nonmaleficence, and, at least in much of the Western world, autonomy. Therapists should help and not hurt. Patients should be able to decide what treatments to undertake. The more closely e-therapy develops in accordance with these basic ethical values, the more widely it will be accepted. Guidelines can help both the therapist and the patient. The therapist will have a better idea of how to treat the patient, and the patient will have a better idea of how to expect to be treated.

Ethical guidelines have long existed for the provision of mental health services in person. Traditionally, they have been specific to particular disciplines in particular countries. For example, the American Psychiatric Association (APA, 2001) has annotated the seven principles of the American Medical Association (AMA), and the American Psychological Association Ethics Committee has issued its own detailed principles (1992). Some degree of international collaboration does, however, take place. The Danish, Norwegian, and Swedish psychological associations, for example, share principles for Nordic psychologists (Dansk Psykolog Forening, 2000; Norsk Psykologforening, 1998; Sveriges Psykologförbund, 1998).

Guidelines have been developed for the provision of health information online (Asmonga, 2000; Boyer, Selby, Scherrer, & Appel, 1998; Health on the Net Foundation, 1997; Hi-Ethics, Inc., 2000; Internet Healthcare Coalition [IHC], 2000). Providing treatment is, however, more controversial than providing information. Some innovations are first considered outlandish, later questionable, and finally acceptable. Others are never accepted; it is "survival of the fittest" in health care.

The potential drawbacks of e-therapy have long been recognized (Hughes, 2000; Robson & Robson, 2000). Methods of communicating emotions over the Internet are very basic. The therapist may be unaware of conditions or cultural issues that affect the patient. How does a therapist become qualified in e-therapy?

Appreciating, let alone checking, the qualifications of the therapist may be difficult. A person who is unlicensed may promote him- or herself as competent. It may be important for the therapist to determine whether the patient is a minor. Screening of patients for suitability for e-therapy may be inadequate. The therapist has no way of knowing who is in the room with the patient. While communicating with the therapist, the patient may be interrupted—or, if in a public area, observed—by others. Messages may be intercepted. The patient may be in a state of emotional distress and unable to understand security issues. The patient may accidentally send a message to someone else meant for the therapist (or vice versa). Patients may use their office computer for e-therapy, unaware that their employer has a right to read all employee e-mail. Following a duty-to-warn mandate may be difficult if the patient has given no identifying information. Technical failures may make reliability difficult to achieve. It may not be possible to assist the patient in locating local support. It may be easier for abusive therapists to hide their intentions—and even their identity. It may be more difficult for the patient to access formal complaint procedures and for the exploitative therapist to be traced by authorities. A path through these many ethical shoals has been slower to emerge.

In 1996, Shapiro and Schulman proposed an ethics standard stating that "e-mail facilitated therapeutic communication" should be discouraged except for general questions, should not take place repeatedly between the same therapist and patient, and therefore would not create a therapist–patient relationship. In 1997, the American Psychological Association Ethics Committee stated that therapists should follow the same guidelines when delivering services online as they do in person. The National Board for Certified Counselors (Bloom, 1998; NBCC, 1999) and the American Counseling Association (1999) developed standards specifically for online counseling, and the Australian Psychological Society (APS, 1999) considered both educational and clinical online services. All of these standards were synthesized and expanded on to produce the suggested principles detailed in the next section.

The Suggested Principles

The Psychiatric Society for Informatics (PSI) and the International Society for Mental Health Online (ISMHO) are organizations with a special interest in online mental health issues. The former was founded in May 1995 and is composed exclusively of psychiatrists. The latter was founded in August 1997 and is composed mostly of clinical psychologists, but includes mental health professionals of other disciplines and also laypersons.

Early in its existence, ISMHO formed "Committee A" to develop guidelines for informational mental health Web sites. In July 1998, the committee's mission was broadened to include the development of these principles. In September 1998, the committee was opened to members of PSI.[2]

The goal of the committee was to guide both the therapists who provide such services and the patients who receive them. The principles were to be broad enough to apply to the entire continuum of clinical mental health services that might be provided online, from e-mail exchanged between office sessions to

---

[2] The members of the joint International Society for Mental Health Online/Psychiatric Society for Informatics "Committee A" were Martha Ainsworth (co-chair), Michael Fenichel, Denis Franklin, John Greist, John Grohol, Leonard Holmes, Robert Hsiung (co-chair), Martin Kesselman, Peggy Kirk, Judy Kraybill, Russell Lim, Roger Park-Cunningham, Richard N. Rosenthal, Jeanne N. Rust, Gary Stofle, Nancy Tice, Giovanni Torello, Mark Vardell, and Willadene Walker-Schmucker.

real-time videoconferencing between therapists and patients who never met in person. The principles were also to be general enough to have international application.

The development of these principles was conducted completely online. An electronic mailing list was created for the committee. The author drafted an initial set of principles, based on four existing sets of guidelines (American Psychological Association Ethics Committee, 1997; Health on the Net Foundation, 1997; Kane & Sands, 1998; National Board for Certified Counselors, 1999) and work of his own (Hsiung, 1999a, 1999b), and revised it as discussion progressed.

On September 7, 1999, the principles were put before the ISMHO and PSI memberships (again, online). There was wider discussion and further revision. An online ISMHO vote, concluded on January 9, 2000, was unanimous in favor of endorsement, and PSI endorsed the principles (with other revisions) when it met in person on May 13, 2000.

Since then, few additional changes have been made. "Regulatory" issues were considered subsumed under "legal" ones, the possibility that patients might feel safer online was added, "competence" was broadened to include not just the types of problems addressed but also the use of the Internet to address them, "requirements to practice" were specified as "legal," third-party coverage was mentioned, and minor changes in wording were made.

These principles have been published online (ISMHO & PSI, 2000a, 2000b), reported on ("Ground Rules for Online Services," 2000), and published in print (Hsiung, 2001). Below is the current version, 3.16.intermed (10/6/00).

Suggested Principles of Professional Ethics for the Online Provision of Mental Health Services

A. INFORMED CONSENT
Informed consent is one of the foundations of ethical health care today. Before the patient consents to receive online mental health services, he or she should be informed about the process, the therapist, the potential risks and benefits, safeguards, and alternatives.

1. Process
   a. Possible misunderstandings
      The patient should be informed that when interacting online with the therapist, less information about each may be available to the other, so misunderstandings may be more likely. With text-based modalities such as email, nonverbal cues are relatively lacking, and even with videoconferencing, bandwidth is limited.

   b. Turnaround time

One issue specific to the provision of mental health services using asynchronous (not in "real time") communication is that of turnaround time. The patient should be informed of how soon after sending an e-mail, for example, he or she may expect a response.

   c. Privacy of the therapist

Privacy is more of an issue online than in person. The therapist has a right to his or her privacy and may wish to restrict the use of any copies or recordings the patient makes of their communications. See also the below on the confidentiality of the patient.

2. Therapist

When the patient and the therapist do not meet in person, the patient may be less able to assess the therapist and to decide whether or not to enter into a treatment relationship with him or her.

   a. Name

The patient should be informed of the name of the therapist. The use of pseudonyms is common online, but is insufficient in a clinical context.

   b. Qualifications and how to confirm them

The patient should be informed of the qualifications (for example, having a degree or being licensed, certified, or registered) of the therapist. The therapist may also wish to provide supplemental information such as areas of special training or experience. So that the patient can confirm the qualifications, the therapist should provide the telephone numbers or web page URLs of the relevant organizations.

3. Potential benefits

The patient should be informed of the potential benefits of receiving mental health services online. This includes both the circumstances in which the therapist considers online mental health services appropriate and the possible advantages of providing those services online. An example of the latter is that the patient might feel safer and therefore less inhibited.

4. Potential risks

The patient should be informed of the potential risks of receiving mental health services online, for example, that misunderstandings might interfere with evaluation or treatment or that confidentiality might be breached.

5. Safeguards

The patient should be informed of safeguards (such as the use of encryption) that are taken by the therapist and could be taken by himself or herself against the potential risks. Extra safeguards should be considered when family members, students, library patrons, etc., share a computer.

6. Alternatives

The patient should be informed of alternatives to receiving mental health services online.

7. Proxies

Some patients are not in a position to consent themselves to receive mental health services. In those cases, consent should be obtained from a parent, legal guardian, or other authorized party—and the identity of that party should be verified.

B. STANDARD OPERATING PROCEDURE

The mental health professions have evolved a standard service delivery framework. When treatment is provided online, that framework need not—indeed, should not—be discarded.

1. Competence

The therapist should remain within the boundaries of competence determined by his or her education and training, both in regard to the types of problems addressed and the online provision of services.

2. Legal requirements to practice

The therapist should meet any legal requirements (for example, have a degree or be licensed, certified, or registered) to provide mental health services where he or she is located. In fact, the legal requirements where the patient is located may also need to be met for it to be legal to provide services to that patient. See also the above on qualifications.

3. Structure of the online services

The therapist and the patient should agree on the frequency and mode of communication, the method for determining the fee, the estimated total cost to the patient (third-party coverage may or may not apply), the payment procedure, etc.

4. Evaluation

The therapist should adequately evaluate the patient when providing any mental health services online. The patient should understand that that evaluation could potentially be helped or hindered by communicating online.

5. Multiple treatment providers

When the patient receives mental health services from others at the same time, either online or in person, the therapist should carefully consider the potential effects of his or her interventions in the overall treatment context.

6. Confidentiality of the patient

The confidentiality of the patient should be protected. Information about the patient should be released only with his or her permission. The patient should be informed of any exceptions to this general rule.

7. Records

The therapist should maintain records of the services provided. If those records include copies or recordings of communications with the patient, the patient should be informed.

8. Existing guidelines

The therapist should of course follow the laws and other existing guidelines (such as those of professional organizations) that apply to him or her.

C. EMERGENCIES

When mental health services are provided online, the therapist can be a great distance from the patient. This may limit the ability to respond to an emergency.

1. Procedures

The procedures to follow in an emergency should be discussed. These procedures should address the possibility that the therapist might not immediately receive an online communication (perhaps because of technical problems) and might include trying to call the therapist, an answering service, or a local backup.

2. Local backup

When the therapist and the patient are in fact geographically separated, the therapist should identify and obtain the telephone number of a qualified local health care provider. A local backup who already knows the patient, such as his or her primary care physician, may be preferable.

Terminology

The committee referred to these principles as "suggested" because its goal was to guide and educate, not to impose or regulate. There was some debate over the terms for the provider and recipient of services. *Provider* and *recipient* themselves seemed too bureaucratic. ISMHO endorsed *counselor* and *client*, and PSI endorsed *psychiatrist* and *patient*. Here, an intermediate terminology—*therapist* and *patient*—is used.

A contentious question was "where" e-therapy was provided. Was it where the therapist or the patient was located? Some have argued that it was "in cyberspace"! A more productive way to frame the issue was in terms of legal requirements to practice. The therapist should meet any legal requirements where he or she is located, but may also need to meet the legal requirements where the patient is located. One rationale is that it is the authorities there who have the responsibility of protecting the patient. The more general *legal requirements to practice* was preferred over the more specific *license* because being licensed is a requirement for psychiatrists and clinical psychologists throughout the United States, but is not, for example, for pastoral counselors in 10 states or for clinical psychologists in Australia or Italy.

Estimated total cost to the patient was specified under *structure of the online services* because it was considered inadequate, for example, to inform the patient of a per-minute or per-word rate without at least a range of how many minutes or words would typically be billed. Finally, the local backup was referred to as a *provider* rather than as a *clinician* so that a hospital emergency room or other service could serve that function.

The following comments reflect the views of the author and not necessarily those of other members of Committee A.

Limitations

These principles were developed by a small self-selected group that consisted primarily of psychiatrists and clinical psychologists in the United States. This might have limited its perspective. In addition, the very undertaking of the development of these principles could be taken to imply an underlying bias in favor of e-therapy.

Other limitations stem from the scope of these principles. They are ethical, as opposed to clinical or legal, in nature. Adequately evaluating the patient is an ethical issue, but how to evaluate a particular patient online—and whether doing so is even possible—is a clinical question. Simply having someone click an "impotence" button on a Web page to be prescribed sildenafil (Viagra) would, however, clearly be inadequate. Meeting requirements to practice is an ethical issue, but what specific requirements need to be met given a particular therapist and a particular patient is a legal question (and varies depending on the discipline and jurisdiction, and may change over time). Whether a given service is a clinical one (i.e., constitutes e-therapy) is another legal question. There is currently no consensus regarding the meaning of terms like *consultation*—in some cases it might be a clinical service, in other cases, not. Maintaining records of services provided is a ethical issue, but the form in which to maintain them (electronic or paper, transcripts or summaries, etc.) is an administrative question.

These are principles, not a blueprint. It remains to be determined how to put them into practice given particular therapists, patients, and practice settings. Research will need to be conducted, experience will need to be gained, and clinical judgment will need to be applied. Some issues remain unresolved. First, verifying the identity of a proxy is not a simple matter; the signature of a parent or guardian could be requested, but could easily be forged. Second, a person who is unlicensed could promote him- or herself as competent not by claiming false credentials, but by claiming the actual credentials of a qualified therapist by posing as that person ("stealing" the therapist's identity). That may occur offline as well. Third, there is the question of how or even whether to work with a patient who insists on anonymity.

What about enforcement? These principles were designed to guide, to influence through education. The clearer therapists are about what they should provide and patients are about they should expect, the higher the standard of care will be. These principles could, however, be enforced. Professional organizations such as ISMHO and PSI—or, on a larger scale, the American Psychiatric Association, the American Psychological Association, the National Association of Social Workers, and so on—could endorse some or all of these principles and require compliance as a condition of membership (i.e., discipline members who violate them). Similarly, government agencies could require compliance as a condition of licensure, certification, registration, and so on. Finally, courts could look to these principles for guidance in legal proceedings. Boulding discussed the complementary nature of self-regulation and legal enforcement (2000).

Tradeoffs

The Internet is a double-edged sword. The patient may feel safer and less inhibited, and therefore be more revealing online than in person. On the other hand, visual, auditory, and olfactory channels of information are at best limited, so the therapist has less data with which to work. In some cases, the net effect will be positive; in others, negative. Which are which, and how to work with each, are clinical questions.

Using text-based modalities such as e-mail makes it easier to record communications. Having a transcript to refer to can help the patient—and provide additional incentive for the therapist to provide good care (Murphy & Mitchell,

1998)—but it also makes it easier for the patient to violate the privacy of the therapist by releasing that text to others.

Finally, the Internet gives each therapist access to more patients and each patient access to more therapists. Efficiency should result from this freer "market." However, regulatory bodies still need to be able to protect patients. The market should not be so free that quacks can make fraudulent claims and harm patients with impunity.

Other Guidelines

King and Moreggi (1998) had concerns about the lack of guidelines and a governing body, the possible inappropriateness of e-therapy for certain problems, and the potential for misdiagnosis. They observed that "the Internet provides an arena where an individual can create a personality character, not unlike a writer imagining the main character in his new novel" (p. 101). To some extent, however, we all create our characters, and "as if" pseudoaffectivity was described long before the Internet (Deutsch, 1942). King and Moreggi also recommended that informed consent be obtained, local backup be available, and referrals to appropriate psychoeducational material online be made.

Holmes (1998) felt therapists were obligated to inform potential patients of risks to confidentiality, and to "do what they can" to keep their patients safe if, for example, they were suicidal. He acknowledged, however, that this would be possible only to the extent that identifying information had been supplied.

Rodriguez (1999) focused on providing public information by responding to questions through Web sites. However, she explicitly distinguished that from individual counseling.

The American Counseling Association (ACA) Ethical Standards for Internet Online Counseling (1999) overlap with these suggested principles on 16 points. They also cover four points these suggested principles do not: identifying the patient, contacting the patient in an emergency, informing the patient of how long records are kept, and seeking appropriate legal and technical assistance in developing e-therapy services.

Rosik and Brown (2001) proposed a number of specific measures to promote ethical practice. Encryption should be used whenever communicating with or about a patient by e-mail, unless the patient has explicitly waived that option. The patient should be informed that confidential or sensitive information should not be sent via office e-mail, even with encryption. All patient-related e-mail should contain a notice that the message is confidential. When treatment teams are involved, all staff members should have their own e-mail address. Consent should be in written form and obtained prior to using e-mail. Technology-specific disclosures should include: the lack of confidentiality guarantees; the inclusion of electronically transmitted information in the record; how electronic records will be stored and who will have access to them; the differences between e- and traditional therapy; the advantages, disadvantages, and experimental nature of e-therapy; normal response times; ways to confirm the therapist's identity and qualifications; security measures in place; and the probable right of a parent to the records of a child who is a minor. Responses should be written by the therapist. Arrangements during the therapist's absences should be made. The patient should be notified of any prohibited topics. The therapist should consider getting training and education in e-therapy. The therapist should have a plan for handling emergencies and technical failures. If the therapist advertises e-therapy services, he or she should fully describe them.

Further Development

These principles are a work in progress—as e-therapy itself is still evolving. Additional input has been and continues to be sought from other interested parties (including readers of this chapter). In particular, data regarding the relevance and utility of these principles in practice will be essential. The author has created a message board for discussion of "distance" mental health services, including these principles. As of this writing, there have been 68 posts to the board, 36 from members of Committee A. There has been technical discussion, for example, about how to allow users to confirm a credential by simply clicking a button, about different methods of encryption, and so on. There has also been discussion about more general issues such as the reluctance of "mainstream" physicians to use the Internet to communicate with patients. No further revisions of the principles have yet been proposed or made.

Conclusions

Traditional principles of professional ethics can be extended to e-therapy. The wheel does not need to be reinvented, although it does need to be modified for this new terrain.

Comprehensive principles of professional ethics can be developed by groups that cross disciplinary and national boundaries. Although there are, of course, differences among the traditions and current practices of different professionals in different countries, ethical principles are derived from cultural values, and principles derived from values common to a number of cultures should be applicable in those cultures.

Productive collaboration can take place entirely online. Not having to meet at the same place at the same time allows more people to be involved and a wider range of perspectives to be represented.

That these guiding principles were agreed on also suggests that consensus regarding binding principles might be reached, and therefore that online therapists have the potential to regulate themselves.

These principles should help guide both the therapists who provide and the patients who receive e-therapy. These individuals will then be able to benefit from the opportunities of this new treatment modality while avoiding its dangers, and others will then be reassured that e-therapy can be conducted ethically. To paraphrase King and Moreggi (1998), e-therapy may be controversial today but commonplace tomorrow.

Another Scenario

Therapist B, in California, decides to diversify into e-therapy. He is aware of the ISMHO/PSI guidelines and creates a virtual shingle: "Therapy Services Online, Inc. Get help by secure real-time chat. Therapist B, Ph.D. Licensed in California. E-mail now for more information, but keep in mind that e-mail may be intercepted by hackers, read by employers, or misunderstood by the recipient. Please therefore think twice about what you say, how you say it, and where you say it from." Patient B sees Therapist A's Web page, but doesn't see Therapist A's name or qualifications and moves on. Next, he sees Therapist B's Web page. Heeding its advice, he sends an e-mail: "There's something I'm concerned about, and I wonder if you can help me with it. Can we chat to discuss this further?" He starts corresponding with other e-therapists, too.

Therapist B and Patient B have a chat meeting, and Therapist B says he charges $100/hour spent chatting or responding to e-mail. Patient B accepts, but makes a mental note not to e-mail Therapist B unnecessarily. Therapist B says Patient B can expect e-mail to be responded to within 12 hours. Therapist B asks if Patient B has a primary care physician. Patient B does, Doctor B, and gives Therapist B her name and telephone number. Therapist B instructs Patient B to call Doctor B if he can't contact Therapist B in an emergency.

They start having chat meetings. Patient B tells Therapist B about his passionate feelings for his boss's wife. Therapist B asks about other concurrent therapy relationships, and Patient B tells him about the other e-therapists. Therapist B explains how too many cooks can spoil the broth, and Patient B accepts that and terminates with the others. Therapist B asks what Patient B had been discussing with them, and Patient B says one issue was his feelings of commitment to his wife. They discuss both his satisfactions and dissatisfactions in his marriage.

To fill Therapist B in on the history of his affair, Patient B e-mails him entries from his diary. Not wanting to pay Therapist B to go through irrelevant material, Patient B is selective about what he sends. Therapist B spends 30 minutes reviewing and commenting on the diary entries and enters that time into his automatic billing software.

Therapist B is then unexpectedly called away. The boss's wife calls Patient B at home and gives him an ultimatum.

Patient B immediately sends Therapist B an e-mail, but, aware of the risks of using his home computer, first unchecks the default "save a copy" feature. Not getting a response within 12 hours, he decides Therapist B must be having technical problems and calls Doctor B, as previously discussed. Doctor B advises him not to take any lithium and prescribes a benzodiazepine instead. Feeling more relaxed, Patient B reflects on his situation and considers his options. Therapist B's automatic billing service sends an e-mail bill to him for the month's chat sessions plus $50 for dealing with the diary entries. Patient B grumbles to himself about the extra charge, but feels confident that he will find his way and looks forward to continuing to work with Therapist B when they are able to connect again.

References

American Counseling Association. (1999). *Ethical standards for Internet online counseling* [Online]. Available: www.counseling.org/gc/cybertx.htm

American Psychiatric Association. (2001). *Principles of medical ethics with annotations especially applicable to psychiatry* [Online]. Available: www.psych.org/apa_members/medicalethics2001_42001.cfm

American Psychological Association Ethics Committee. (1992). Ethical principles of psychologists and code of conduct. *American Psychologist, 47*(12), 1597–1611 [Online]. Available: www.apa.org/ethics/code.html

American Psychological Association Ethics Committee. (1997). *Services by telephone, tele-conferencing, and Internet* [Online]. Available: www.apa.org/ethics/stmnt01.html

Asmonga, D. D. (2000). IHC eyes E-health Code of Ethics. *Journal of Ahima, 71*(6), 14–6.

Australian Psychological Society. (1999). *Considerations for psychologists providing services on the Internet* [Online]. Available: faps.psychsociety.com.au/about/internet.pdf

Bloom, J. W. (1998). The ethical practice of webcounseling. *British Journal of Guidance & Counselling, 26*(1), 53–59.

Boulding, M. E. (2000). Self-regulation: Who needs it? *Health Affairs, 19*(6), 132–139.

Boyer, C., Selby, M., Scherrer, J. R., & Appel, R. D. (1998). The Health on the Net code of conduct for medical and health websites. *Computers in Biology & Medicine, 28*(5), 603–610.

Dansk Psykolog Forening. (2000). *Etiske principper for nordiske psykologer* [Online]. Available: www.dp.dk/Menu.asp?id=152

Deutsch, H. (1942). Some forms of emotional disturbance and their relationship to schizophrenia. *Psychoanalytic Quarterly, 11*, 301–321.

Ground rules for online services. (2000). *Behavioral Healthcare Tomorrow, 9*(2), 22–25.

Health on the Net Foundation. (1997). *Health on the Net code of conduct (HONcode) for medical and health websites* [Online]. Available: www.hon.ch/HONcode/Conduct.html

Hi-Ethics, Inc. (2000). *Ethical principles for offering Internet health services to consumers* [Online]. Available: www.hiethics.com/Principles/index.asp

Holmes, L. G. (1998). Delivering mental health services on-line: Current issues. *Cyberpsychology & Behavior, 1*(1), 19–24.

Hsiung, R. C. (1999a, May). *Clinical use of the Internet: Some suggestions.* Paper presented at the meeting of the American Psychiatric Association, Washington, DC.

Hsiung, R. C. (1999b, August). *Electronic communication with clients.* Paper presented at the meeting of the American Psychological Association, Boston, MA.

Hsiung, R. C. (2001). Suggested principles of professional ethics for the online provision of mental health services. *Telemedicine Journal and E-Health, 7*(1), 39–45.

Hughes, R. S. (2000). Cybercounseling and regulations: Quagmire or quest? In J. W. Bloom & G. R. Walz (Eds.), *Cybercounseling and cyberlearning: Strategies and resources for the millennium* (pp. 321–338). Alexandria, VA: American Counseling Association.

International Society for Mental Health Online & Psychiatric Society for Informatics. (2000a). *ISMHO/PSI suggested principles of professional ethics for the online provision of mental health services* [Online]. Available: www.ismho.org/suggestions.html

International Society for Mental Health Online & Psychiatric Society for Informatics. (2000b). *ISMHO/PSI suggested principles of professional ethics for the online provision of mental health services* [Online]. Available: www.dr-bob.org/psi/suggestions.3.13.html

Internet Healthcare Coalition. (2000). *eHealth code of ethics* [Online]. Available: www.ihealthcoalition.org/ethics/ehealthcode0524.html

Kane, B., & Sands, D. Z. (1998). Guidelines for the clinical use of electronic mail with patients. *Journal of the American Medical Informatics Association, 5*(1), 104–111.

King, S. A., & Moreggi, D. (1998). Internet therapy and self-help groups—the pros and cons. In J. Gackenbach (Ed.), *Psychology and the Internet: Intrapersonal, interpersonal, and transpersonal implications* (pp. 77–109). San Diego, CA: Academic Press.

Murphy, L. J., & Mitchell, D. L. (1998). When writing helps to heal: E-mail as therapy. *British Journal of Guidance & Counselling, 26*(1), 21–32.

National Board for Certified Counselors (NBCC) (1999). *Standards for the ethical practice of webcounseling* [Online]. Available: www.nbcc.org/ethics/wcstandards.htm

Norsk Psykologforening. (1998). *Etiske prinsipper for nordiske psykologer* [Online]. Available: www.psykol.no/npf_organisasjon/etiske_prinsipper.html

Robson, D., & Robson, M. (2000). Ethical issues in Internet counselling. *Counselling Psychology Quarterly, 13*(3), 249–257.

Rodriguez, J. C. (1999). Legal, ethical, and professional issues to consider when communicating via the Internet: A suggested response model and policy. *Journal of the American Dietetic Association, 99*(11), 1428–1432.

Rosik, C. H., & Brown, R. K. (2001). Professional use of the Internet: Legal and ethical issues in a member care environment. *Journal of Psychology & Theology, 29*(2), 106–120.

Shapiro, D. E., & Schulman C. E. (1996). Ethical and legal issues in e-mail therapy. *Ethics and Behavior, 6,* 107–124.

Sveriges Psykologförbund. (1998). *Yrkesetiska principer för psykologer i norden* [Online]. Available: www.psykologforbundet.se/etik.html#del1

8

The Legal Implications of E-Therapy[1]

Nicolas P. Terry

THE GROWTH OF e-health—the utilization of technology to deliver or to improve the delivery of health care services—implicates the familiar triad of quality, access, and cost. In the mental health arena, these competing concerns are highlighted by scope of practice issues involving psychiatrists, psychologists, and other counselors and a recent history of limited reimbursement for traditional mental health services. This chapter describes the complex bundle of products and services that will impact technologically mediated mental health care, and highlights how it challenges our traditional regulatory approaches, liability systems, and ethical constructs.

E-Health, E-Therapy, and Telepsychiatry

Many clinicians and agencies are involved in a well-established form of e-therapy—consultation with geographically remote colleagues. This type of service, a subset of telemedicine, is referred to herein as *telepsychiatry*. Telepsychiatry is legally and ethically uncontentious; however, it remains a small part of the burgeoning practice of e-therapy.

In addition to traditional telemedicine, e-health business-to-business (B2B) services and transactions already include robust continuing professional education (Greene, 2001), publishing, and procurement. Of growing importance,

---

[1]Based in part on a speech delivered at the invitation of the American Psychiatric Association Council on Psychiatry and Law and Committee on Information Technology, May 8, 2001, New Orleans.

however, are the "backend" or administrative services that will come to dominate the e-health industry. These include billing, insurance reimbursement, and prescription fulfillment systems.

Vertical portals, relatively simple patient advice sites, and support groups were the original business-to-consumer (B2C) e-health services. The portal segment has experienced a period of rapid consolidation, leaving WebMD as the dominant player with 4.4 million discrete visitors per month—twice as many as the next largest ("Top Health Care," 2001). Despite this, sophisticated new services continue to enter the e-health market. Many of these new services operate as "infomediaries." Examples include group-buying services, whose goal is to reduce the costs of treatment, pharmaceuticals, or insurance; Web sites that match patients and clinical trials; and, most controversially, treatment auctions. Arriving on their heels are increasingly sophisticated consumer product and Web-service hybrids, such as Web-connected medical appliances or devices (e.g., Matsushita, 2001) that will enable remote diagnosis, monitoring, and even treatment.

In e-health, the industry message is resolutely upbeat. Examples include Microsoft telling consumers that, with its new e-health systems, "the patient is definitely in charge" (Microsoft, 2000); or the American Medical Association (AMA) introducing products such as Medem (www.medem.com), its Web site hosting service for physicians, with the snappy tag line "Finding solutions to the e-health puzzle: AMA puts the pieces together for you and your patients" (American Medical Association, 2001c). The latest AMA survey suggests this industry confidence is rubbing off on doctors ("AMA Survey," 2001). Although the proportion of physicians having a Web site has leveled off, the survey discloses significant increases in physician use of the Web for research and as a resource for patient education. Furthermore, roughly one quarter of online physicians communicate with their patients via e-mail. Perhaps less encouraging is a developing pattern of increased consumer use of online health care information coupled with a decline in those users' satisfaction with that information (Landro, 2000).

In late 2001, e-therapy remained dominated by traditional telepsychiatry, which was typically performed via telephone or, increasingly, videoconferencing. These forms of telemedicine feature integrated, frequently community-based approaches to remote care. Far less controversial than the emerging products, telepsychiatry has already been the subject of extensive study and comment (e.g., American Psychiatric Association, 1998). Almost by definition, these intrastate programs seldom implicate licensure issues. Additionally, as state initiatives, they are less likely to be investigated by other state bodies such as medical disciplinary boards. The relative importance of such programs is a function of the amount of public funding, and President Bush's proposed budget for fiscal year 2002 may have been a predictor of deep cuts in the budget of the Office for the Advancement of Telehealth (OAT) (telehealth.hrsa.gov).

In contrast to psychiatrists' limited adoption of more aggressive forms of e-health, psychologists and other counselors are embracing the latest technologies and comprehending patient use patterns. These other professionals increasingly offer B2C e-therapy. Even relatively unscientific forays into the space using Web search engines disclose a significantly increasing number of entries for "Mental Health" and particularly strong increases for what are generically labeled as "Counseling Services" (Google, August 21, 2000 vs. April 25, 2001). Sites run by psychiatrists and psychologists are considerably less plentiful than those run by other counselors. Many B2C e-therapy sites have a somewhat transitory existence, as they appear and then disappear from the Web. Sites run by psychiatrists and psychologists tend to be less aggressive in their adoption of technological intermediation (both synchronous and asynchronous) than those run by other counselors (e.g., videoShrink, www.videoshrink.com; here2listen.com, www.here2listen.com; We Ain't Freud, www.weaintfreud.com).

Overall, psychiatrists have assumed a low profile on the Web. There are comparatively few publicly accessible sites operated by individual psychiatrists, although some are appearing on Medem (e.g., www.foresthillspsych. medem.com). WebMD (www.webmd.com) lists a large number of psychiatrists, but an insignificant percentage of the profession. Further, of those listed by WebMD few earn the apparent distinction of being labeled as a "WebMD Participating Physician," and only an insignificant number link their entries to Web pages or list e-mail addresses.

The popular press has noted that "Internet mental-health services are growing rapidly, but there's no solid evidence that good therapy can be done on line" (Elias, 2000). Notwithstanding, the shift toward B2C e-therapy is as unrelenting as the parallel phenomena seen elsewhere in e-commerce. Various forces— such as perceived consumer demand and a belief that reimbursement is likely— may conspire to accelerate this trend. Although controversial, dialogue-based health care services, such as psychotherapy, are viewed as naturals for technological mediation.

Structural, Legal, and Ethical Implications

Routine delivery of health care over the Web will involve relationships that are fundamentally different from any that have evolved in modern health care delivery. Although the way U.S. health care is financed has changed dramatically over the last few decades, the shifts from fee-for-service to managed care and from independent to partially or fully integrated systems have done little to change the underlying structure of a health delivery system that controls access by way of a small number of predetermined points of entry (e.g., primary care physicians) and dictates patient progress through relatively linear, often hierarchical, structures. As I have noted:

> Web and attendant e-commerce phenomena are irretrievably at odds with the traditional structure and hence legal regulation of health delivery. E-health delivers healthcare information, diagnosis, treatment, care, and prescribing of drugs in a nonlinear, nonhierarchical manner that encourages patients to "enter" the system at an infinite number of points, thus defying current regulatory constructs. Similarly, e-commerce fundamentals such as disintermediation and disaggregation result in medical information being delivered through unfamiliar channels, creating immensely difficult questions for health lawyers. (Terry, 2000b, p. 605)

New channels herald the entry of new, possibly heretofore unregulated entities into the health care delivery arena. Additionally, e-health business models that feature anonymity and lack physicality are particularly challenging to traditional state-based legal regulatory systems. Liability systems are also upset by new technologies or business models that exploit Web business strategies such as disaggregation or disintermediation that result in new provider–consumer relationships.

Ethical structures are equally challenged. Emanuel and Dubler (1995), with their cautionary tale of the six Cs (choice, competence, communication, compassion, continuity, and [no] conflict of interest), have noted the difficulties of transferring the core tenets of the physician–patient relationship to the more industrialized, commercialized world of managed care. But e-health poses even more difficult problems. In that context, I have suggested that:

> Choice and communication (aided by the promise of reducing administrative costs from the healthcare delivery system) should dramatically improve access. Yet, e-health's lack of physicality, its depersonalization, anonymity, and even coldness challenge usual conceptions of competence and compassion. Further, multipoint entry into the delivery system makes continuity difficult to achieve, while health advice sites based on e-commerce paradigms involve considerable conflicts of interest. Finally, e-health marketing practices and privacy concerns frequently seem to involve the commodification of patients and patient data. (Terry, 2001a)

It must also be appreciated that legal and ethical constraints will overlap and together may be severely tested when dealing with Web issues. For example, there is a recurring conflict-of-interest issue relating to the placement of advertisements, particularly for pharmaceuticals, on medical advice sites. These ethically suspect placements and other injudicious links could implicate Medicare and Medicaid kickback prohibitions (42 USC § 1320a-7b; 42 USC § 1395nn) or adversely affect an institution's tax exempt status ("Request for Comments," 2000; Terry, 2001b).

Four general sets of legal issues are affected by the growth of e-therapy: regulation, including licensure and prescribing; the therapist–patient relationship, including identification and consent; quality of care, including the impact of technology on traditional health care delivery; and security and privacy. These are examined in the sections that follow.

Regulatory Issues

The regulation of cyberspace activities is severely challenged by a federal system that allocates some responsibilities to federal authorities and some to state authorities. Although the federal government controls the health purse and the approval and marketing of prescription drugs, the states traditionally have regulated doctors and pharmacists, both directly through licensure systems and indirectly through malpractice-based quality of care. Problems are exacerbated when activities are highly regulated at both federal and state levels, as is the case with health care. This dynamic is further complicated by the practicalities of the federal government enforcing essentially state-regulated issues, as is the case with unlicensed prescribing.

Agencies may not be adequately legally empowered to regulate emergent business activities. For example, the Federal Trade Commission (FTC) has been seriously hampered in its efforts to protect consumer privacy on the Internet by a legislative mandate that requires the agency to demonstrate "unfair or deceptive acts or practices in or affecting commerce" [15 USC § 45(a)(1)]. This requirement makes those who breach their own privacy policies more susceptible to action than those who have no privacy policies at all.

Even within a single state, multiple agencies may be involved. For example, Michigan's Bureau of Health Services (www.cis.state.mi.us/bhser/lic/occup.htm) has separate licensing boards for medical doctors, psychologists, licensed professional counselors, and marriage and family therapists. It is through these boards that new e-therapy practice models must navigate, and within this regulatory setting that they must emerge and mature. The more aggressive forms of e-therapy (primarily B2C) must be assessed for their legal implications within this confusing and gap-laden regulatory environment.

Licensure

In the absence of national licensure and with few state reciprocity policies, the lawful practice of e-therapy is considerably hampered by state licensure laws and, equally as important, by the practices of the state boards that investigate and discipline doctors (American Medical Association, 2001a; Silverman, 2000) and other therapists. Although different states apply slightly different verbiage, the key concept is the "practice of medicine," which the states regulate within their borders and which typically consists of:

(a) Holding out one's self to the public within this state as being able to diagnose, treat, prescribe for, palliate, or prevent any human disease, ailment, pain, injury, deformity, or physical or mental condition, whether by the use of drugs, surgery, manipulation, electricity, telemedicine, the interpretation of tests, including primary diagnosis of pathology specimens, images, or photographs, or any physical, mechanical, or other means whatsoever; [or]

(b) Suggesting, recommending, prescribing, or administering any form of treatment, operation, or healing for the intended palliation, relief, or cure of any physical or mental disease, ailment, injury, condition, or defect of any person with the intention of receiving therefor, either directly or indirectly, any fee, gift, or compensation whatsoever. . . . [Colo. Rev. Stat. § 12-36-106(1)]

Analogous provisions apply to nonpsychiatrist therapists.

A growing number of states have added specific telemedicine provisions to their physician-licensing and disciplinary statutes (e.g., Mont. Code Ann. § 37-3-341).[2] These provisions usually apply to telepsychiatry. For example, Arizona defines telemedicine as:

The practice of health care delivery, diagnosis, consultation, treatment and transfer of medical data through interactive audio, video or data communications that occurs in the physical presence of the patient. For the purposes of this article, audio or video communications sent to a health care provider for diagnostic or treatment consultation also constitute telemedicine. [Ariz. Rev. Stat. § 36-3601(2)]

States provide this special definition in order to impose additional regulatory requirements on the practice of telemedicine. For example, some states require that out-of-state physicians apply for specialty-specific telemedicine practice

---

[2] "The legislature now finds that because of technological advances and changing patterns of medical practice, medicine is increasingly being practiced by electronic means across state lines. Although access to technological advances is in the public interest, the legislature also finds that regulation of the practice of medicine across state lines is necessary to protect the public against the unprofessional, improper, unauthorized, and unqualified practice of medicine."

certificates (e.g., Mont. Code Ann. § 37-3-343). Other states mandate additional consent and recordkeeping requirements for telemedicine (e.g., Ariz. Rev. Stat. § 36-3602).

Different geographical and professional e-therapy practice scenarios will be variously impacted by different licensing and disciplinary statutes. The least controversial involves the provision of telepsychiatry services within a single state. Here, we can assume that both the local treatment provider (typically physically accompanying the patient) and the consulting therapist (typically connecting from a remote location via videoconferencing) are licensed within the same state. Very few licensure issues will arise, although there are other important practical, rather than purely legal, considerations impacting the viability of the consulting therapist's work. First, a question may arise as to whether the consultant has satisfied the institutional privileging requirements of the institution into which his or her opinions are being transmitted. Second, there may be an issue as to whether the consultant's malpractice insurance covers the telemedicine consult and whether such a service is reimbursable. Typically, telemedicine-specific regulations are unlikely to apply to purely intrastate activities (e.g., Mont. Code Ann. § 37-3-342). About the only scenario that will interest a state board in a purely intrastate situation is a case of a psychiatrist who has only technologically mediated contact with a patient, yet still prescribes medication for that patient. Some state boards would view that as unprofessional conduct (e.g., Texas State Board, 1999).

The most basic type of interstate telemedicine interaction is the remote consultation. Here, the patient is in State A and is accompanied by his or her local treatment provider, who is licensed in that state. The remote or consulting psychiatrist, located and licensed in State B, is connected by telephone or videoconferencing. The first question that arises is whether the therapist in State B is practicing in State A. Some states hold that the therapist is not. Others have decided that he or she is. For example:

> *A person engaged in the practice of telemedicine is considered to be engaged in the practice of medicine within this state and is subject to the licensure requirements of this article. As used in this section, the "practice of telemedicine" means the use of electronic information and communication technologies to provide health care when distance separates participants and includes one or both of the following: (1) The diagnosis of a patient within this state by a physician located outside this state as a result of the transmission of individual patient data, specimens or other material by electronic or other means from within this state to the physician or his or her agent; or (2) the rendering of treatment to a patient within this state by a physician located outside this state as a result of transmission of individual patient data, specimens or other material by electronic or other means from within this state to the physician or his or her agent. (W. Va. Code § 30-3-13)*

Some then apply a "consulting" or "temporary practice" exception from the requirement of licensure. For example:

> A doctor of medicine or doctor of osteopathy licensed to practice medicine in any state of the United States or the District of Columbia who may be called into this state in order to treat a patient in consultation with a physician licensed to practice medicine in this state shall be allowed the temporary privilege of practicing medicine in this state. This privilege shall be limited to 10 calendar days in a calendar year. (Ala. Code § 34-24-74)

Technologically mediated "consulting" is likely to be governed by specific telemedicine rules in states that have them, although it should be noted that some telemedicine rules only target more technologically sophisticated consults based on, for example, "interactive data communications," and do not extend to phone consults [e.g., Cal. Bus. & Prof. Code § 2290.5(a)].[3] Again, a practical question that arises in this type of situation is whether the consulting therapist's malpractice insurance covers such an arguably out-of-state activity.

The legal situation becomes considerably more controversial in a case in which there is no local treatment provider in the patient's state (i.e., when we move from B2B telepsychiatry to B2C e-therapy). At first glance, the most important question may be whether the therapist in State B, who is remotely treating the patient in State A, is practicing in State A and thus is subject to State A's licensure or specific telemedicine requirements. The therapist generally is not protected by any out-of-state "consultation" provision in the absence of a local treatment provider. There is, however, limited practical likelihood that State A has the resources to track down the out-of-state therapist. Of course, State B may have some interest in controlling the activities of the therapist if they involve practicing in State A without valid malpractice insurance or prescribing in State A without conducting any physical examinations.

Prescribing Medication

In years past, state and federal task forces targeted Internet pharmacies that dispensed drugs without prescriptions (FDA, 2000; MacMillan, 2001a; Posner, 2000; White House, 1999). Only recently have state regulators turned their

---

[3] "(1) For the purposes of this section, 'telemedicine' means the practice of health care delivery, diagnosis, consultation, treatment, transfer of medical data, and education using interactive audio, video, or data communications. Neither a telephone conversation nor an electronic mail message between a health care practitioner and patient constitutes 'telemedicine' for purposes of this section. (2) For purposes of this section, 'interactive' means an audio, video, or data communication involving a real time (synchronous) or near real time (asynchronous) two-way transfer of medical data and information."

attention to physicians who prescribe without first establishing traditional relationships with patients. The Texas State Board of Medical Examiners was one of the first to issue such an official position, stating that:

> It is unprofessional conduct for a physician to initially prescribe any dangerous drugs or controlled substances without first establishing a proper physician–patient relationship. A proper relationship, at a minimum, requires ... (2) establishing a diagnosis through the use of accepted medical practices such as a patient history, mental status exam, physical examination and appropriate diagnostic and laboratory testing.... (Texas State Board, 1999)

Of course, this policy is easier to state than to enforce, because it is extremely difficult to identify and discipline Internet-based prescribing doctors. More recently, however, Texas has sought to attack the problem by focusing again on pharmacies (see below). Still, more traditional enforcement mechanisms will be required to successfully regulate gray-market e-health providers that are "related" to marginally legal online pharmacies (e.g., U.S. Department of Justice, 1999).

Dispensing Medication

Of course, state licensure issues also directly impact pharmacies. Obviously, illegal operations aside, the licensing issues are somewhat defused in pharmacy cases. In part, this is because the industry and its state regulators previously have weathered the storm of mail-order pharmacies, frequently adapting their laws to take account of such cross-border issues (e.g., Ark. Code Ann. § 17-92-401[4]; 225 Ill. Comp. Stat. 85/16a[5]). A proposed change to the Texas pharmacy regulations would require that:

> A pharmacist may not dispense a prescription drug if the pharmacist knows or should have known that the prescription was issued on the basis of an Internet-based or telephonic

---

[4]"Any pharmacy operating outside the state which routinely ships, mails, or delivers in any manner a dispensed legend drug into Arkansas shall hold a pharmacy license issued by the Arkansas State Board of Pharmacy, and that part of the pharmacy operation dispensing the prescription for an Arkansas resident shall abide by Arkansas law and regulations of the board. (1) Any pharmacy operating outside the state which routinely ships, mails, or delivers in any manner a dispensed legend drug into Arkansas shall be required to have on staff in the out-of-state pharmacy an Arkansas-licensed pharmacist, who shall be designated the pharmacist-in-charge for the Arkansas out-of-state pharmacy license."

[5]"The Department shall establish rules and regulations, consistent with the provisions of this Act, governing mail-order pharmacies, including pharmacies providing services via the Internet, which sell, or offer for sale, drugs, medicines, or other pharmaceutical services in this State."

consultation without a valid patient–practitioner relationship. [Tex. Admin. Code §§ 291.34(b)(1)(B), 291.36(e)(2)(A)(ii)]

Such a rule likely would chill responsible pharmacies from filling any such prescriptions. If successful, this too is a model that would be swiftly replicated across the country.

Pharmacy chains are able to comply with multiple licensure requirements far more easily than are individual physicians. The National Association of Boards of Pharmacy (NABP, www.nabp.net) has been successful in setting up a national system for trustmarking pharmacies through its Verified Internet Pharmacy Practice Sites information and verification site (NABP, 1999).[6] Notwithstanding, the federal government continues to work at enforcing pharmaceutical import laws and drafting additional legislation concerning drugs purchased from non-U.S. Web sites and without legitimate prescriptions ("FDA Wants to Ban," 2001; MacMillan, 2001b).

Interpersonal Issues

Creating a Therapist–Patient Relationship

The touchstone "physician–patient relationship" has been at the center of much of our legal and ethical regulation of the medical and even other mental health professions. Medical malpractice law is replete with statements that physicians are not liable for negligence in the absence of a physician–patient relationship. Many courts no longer insist on a rigid, almost contractual, approach, and the concept has become increasingly amorphous. For example, in a case in which a psychiatrist prescribed Quaalude to a patient but allegedly failed to warn her not to drive while under its influence, the court held that the psychiatrist could be liable to a third party injured by the patient in an automobile accident (*Gooden v. Tips*, 1983; see also *Joy v. Eastern Maine Medical Center*, 1987). In addition, it is important to recognize that the physician–patient relationship is not necessarily concomitant with the "practice of medicine" determination utilized by state licensing laws. Thus, in traditional telepsychiatry, the consultative status of the remote therapist may immunize him or her

---

[6] "To be VIPPS certified, a pharmacy must comply with the licensing and inspection requirements of their state and each state to which they dispense pharmaceuticals. In addition, pharmacies displaying the VIPPS seal have demonstrated to NABP compliance with VIPPS criteria including patient rights to privacy, authentication and security of prescription orders, adherence to a recognized quality assurance policy, and provision of meaningful consultation between patients and pharmacists."

from remote disciplinary scrutiny (i.e., licensing requirements), but may not be determinative as to whether he or she has entered into a therapist–patient relationship and triggered common-law practice duties. Notwithstanding, for many of the issues discussed herein, the creation of a therapist–patient relationship will be the *sine qua non* for the imposition of legal constraints on e-therapists.

As Kuszler (2000) pointed out, mere technologically mediated interaction between a patient and an e-therapist would not be sufficient to create a therapist–patient relationship. It should be noted, however, that increasingly the courts look to the understanding of the patient rather than the intention of the therapist. Telephone cases may be somewhat instructive. For example, in *Miller v. Sullivan*, the court stated:

> *The relationship is created when professional services are rendered and accepted for purposes of medical treatment. A telephone call affirmatively advising a prospective patient as to a course of treatment can constitute professional service for the purpose of creating a physician–patient relationship only when the advice, if incorrect, would be actionable. Thus, it must be shown that it was foreseeable that the prospective patient would rely on the advice and that the prospective patient did in fact rely on the advice. (Miller v. Sullivan, 1995)*

Such a patient-oriented test for the necessary relationship creates considerable hazards for professionals who are online, as does the growing trend of courts to leave the question of the existence of a physician–patient relationship for juries to determine (e.g., *Bienz v. Central Suffolk Hospital*, 1990).[7]

Of all the current technologies that can be used to deliver health care services, it is e-mail that has created the most debate as to when and if such communication creates a therapist–patient relationship. It is, of course, no surprise that so many therapists are now using e-mail for patient communication. E-mail is particularly attractive to therapists because it is rich (e.g., facilitating the inclusion of URL references to other resources that the patient should consider) and self-documenting (in that the stored communications create their own "record" on the therapist's computer). It is arguable, however, that e-mail is even more likely than telephone contact to create a therapist–patient relationship. In large part, this is due to the contemporaneous nature of the communication (contact) and the provision of services (therapeutic dialogue). At the very least, it must be concluded that therapists who enter into e-mail communication are at considerable risk of

---

[7] "Whether the physician's giving of advice furnishes a sufficient basis upon which to conclude that an implied physician–patient relationship had arisen is ordinarily a question of fact for the jury."

exposure to the duties that come with the creation of a therapist–patient relationship.

Eysenbach (2000; see also Sands & Bauer, 2001) argued:

> *Physicians may have an ethical responsibility to read their e-mail and to reply by helping the sender to find someone who can respond to their need. While this may not be always possible in practice, every effort should be made to minimize misunderstanding on the part of the patient, raising false hopes or causing potential harm by, for example, replying with a standard message saying that it is impossible to reply to every e-mail.*

Psychiatrists encounter particularly high risks when they reply to unsolicited e-mail. Psychiatrists who have e-mail accounts would be well advised to compose a single "form letter" reply that is always used (and not further personalized for any individual reply; Eysenbach, 2000). This form letter should state the physician's position that he or she does not enter into professional relationships via e-mail, and that the correspondent should contact his or her own physician or, in the case of an emergency, contact emergency services or visit a hospital emergency room.

Within a Therapist–Patient Relationship

Clearly, e-mail can be an attractive and effective adjunct to traditional communication between therapist and patient. In fact, in just a few years it will likely replace most telephone and postal communication between therapist and patient. Even within the context of an established therapist–patient relationship, e-mail and other technologically mediated supplements to traditional care should not be blindly utilized. As Spielberg (1998) urged, therapists should discuss the ramifications of communicating electronically with patients and obtain relevant informed consent to the technological mediation. Some states are already mandating specific consent. For example, an Arizona statute requires that:

> *Before a health care provider delivers health care through telemedicine, the treating health care provider shall obtain verbal or written informed consent from the patient. If the informed consent is obtained verbally, the health care provider shall document the patient's consent on the patient's medical record. [Ariz. Rev. Stat. § 36-3602(A)]*

Such informed consent presumably would involve notifying the patient that e-mail communication is not intrinsically secure. Patients should be warned that "operator error" frequently leads to e-mail being unexpectedly forwarded and so on (not that such errors by therapists would be tolerated legally). The American Medical Informatics Association (AMIA) has cogently argued that the informed consent mechanism also should "provide instructions for when and how to escalate to phone calls and office visits" and "describe security mechanisms in place" (Kane & Sands, 1998). This latter issue is perhaps the most in need of a legal standard. There is a growing consensus that regular, unsecured e-mail should not be used for anything but the most routine of therapist–patient communications (Medem, 2001b), an issue further complicated by the forthcoming Health Insurance Portability and Accountability Act (HIPAA) security regulations (see below).

In e-therapy, the extent to which therapists use and make it easier for their patients to use e-mail may involve particularly difficult judgment calls insofar as they permit the patients to remain anonymous. Spielberg (1998) observed that "e-mail can strengthen the level of intimacy shared between physician and patient, making more accessible their respective private spheres. Patients, otherwise reluctant to raise sensitive topics in person or seeking only a quick opinion between office visits, may find e-mail inviting." This has particular prescience in the context of B2C e-therapy. Therapists likely will adopt digital certificates to authenticate their own identities as licensed health care professionals (e.g., MEDePass, www.medepass.com; VeriSign, 2001). Overall, it is vital that health care professionals become versed in the limits of our new technologies.

Although there are few, if any, legal answers, professional organizations such as the AMIA (Kane & Sands, 1998), the AMA (2001b), the American Psychological Association (APA, 1997), and the International Society for Mental Health Online and the Psychiatric Society for Informatics (ISMHO & PSI, 2000a, 2000b) have all produced valuable guidance for e-therapists that will clearly shape the eventual legal standards.

Technology and Quality of Care in Traditional Practice

Medical Error

Eclipsing even the rise of e-health in the eyes of medical-legal commentators has been the growing concern over medical error. Although previewed by the Harvard Medical Practice Study (Brennan et al., 1991) a decade earlier, the modern impetus for the search for hard data about medical error, its causes, and its cures has been the 2000 Institute of Medicine (IOM) report, "To Err Is

Human" (IOM, 2000).[8] Unfortunately, the tabloid-friendly sound bite that "at least 44,000 Americans die each year as a result of medical errors" (p. 1) has somewhat obscured the report's principle theme that *process* reform (Reason, 2000) is needed to reduce medical error. A subsequent IOM report, "Crossing the Quality Chasm" (IOM, 2001), recommended a massive infusion of technology into our delivery system:

> *Congress, the executive branch, leaders of health care organizations, public and private purchasers, and health care organizations, public and private purchasers, and health informatics associations and vendors should make a renewed national commitment to building an information infrastructure to support health care delivery, consumer health, quality measurement and improvement, public accountability, clinical and health services research, and clinical education. This commitment should lead to the elimination of most handwritten clinical data by the end of the decade. (IOM, 2001, p.17)*

Fueled by technological innovation, even the most traditional psychiatric practice will not be impervious to the e-health revolution. All physicians will interface with sophisticated new systems designed to both reduce backend tasks and improve the quality of medical care. Even in the traditional practice space, technology and quality assurance will become intertwined. First, technology will be used to target medical error and will become an increasingly important component of risk management and quality assurance programs. The average psychiatrist likely will observe this phenomenon in the increased automation of medication (including automated interaction alerts; e.g., Bates et al., 1998) and other (e.g., Tapellini, 2000) systems, frequently using hand-held devices (e.g., Freudenheim, 2001), and will soon find that such systems are being mandated in institutions where he or she is credentialed.

Malpractice

Remarkably, the admissibility of practice guidelines in malpractice cases remains somewhat unsettled (e.g., *Frakes v. Cardiology Consultants*, 1997). Evidence-based medicine (Sackett, Rosenberg, Gray, Haynes, & Richardson, 1996) likely

---

[8] "Preventing errors means designing the health care system at all levels to make it safer. Building safety into processes of care is a more effective way to reduce errors than blaming individuals. . . . The focus must shift from blaming individuals for past errors to a focus on preventing future errors by designing safety into the system. This does not mean that individuals can be careless. People must still be vigilant and held responsible for their actions. But when an error occurs, blaming an individual does little to make the system safer and prevent someone else from committing the same error." (pp. 4–5)

will be one of the cornerstones of a technology-led approach to decrease medical error. Practice guidelines interacting with the sophisticated electronic patient records systems that providers are installing (in part as a response to HIPAA regulations, see below) will form the basis for medical "expert" systems that will almost inevitably lead to real-time quality of care monitoring.

As these proactive risk-avoidance systems are implemented, the natural correlate is that the normative standard of care expected of all therapists and institutions will rise. Beyond systems directly charged with improving quality assurance, other e-health technologies likely will have important, indirect effects on malpractice litigation. For example, the very strongly delineated consent-to-disclosure provisions in the HIPAA privacy regulations [45 CFR § 164.506, particularly § 164.506(b)(4)(i)] likely will influence the way institutions deal with informed consent-related disclosure, almost inevitably increasing its robustness. Similarly, the combination of HIPAA's implicit mandate to providers to switch to electronic patient records (see Mount, Kelman, Smith, & Douglas, 2000), its explicit data integrity requirements ("Notice of a Proposed Rule Making," 1998), and its audit and access provisions likely will lead to an increase in discovered malpractice and a broadening of the defendant pool. Likewise, the more accurate record likely will increase plaintiffs' recovery rates (Terry, 2001c).

Similar to this somewhat "micro" impact of new regulation, e-health will have more "macro" consequences. Its new business models not only will change the way health care is marketed, structured, and delivered, but also will affect the topography of malpractice liability. As Bates and Gawande (2000) pointed out, "The Internet changes the exercise of quality measurement in several ways. First, quality information—including reputation—will be more readily available. Second, consumers will increasingly use it. Third, the Internet provides a low-cost, standard platform that will make it vastly easier for providers to collect quality information and pass it on to others" (p. 104). The liability correlate to this phenomenon is that the e-health defendant pool will be swelled by an increasing number of intermediaries and infomediaries.

Furthermore, as health care institutions increase their marketing presence on the Web and elsewhere, they will stress their own reputations more than those of individual clinicians. Courts already are noticing this trend and seem prepared to adapt malpractice liability rules, which will inevitably lead to institutions replacing clinicians as the default defendants in malpractice suits (e.g., *Kashishian v. Port,* 1992). A similar phenomenon is playing out in the interpretation of liability rules regarding prescription pharmaceuticals. The "old" learned intermediary rule that set up prescribing physicians as the primary defendants in failure to warn cases (e.g., *Tracy v. Merrell Dow Pharmaceuticals,* 1991) has been fatally undercut by the growth of direct-to-consumer (DTC) pharmaceutical advertising ("Direct-to-Consumer Promotion," 1996; "Guidance for Industry," 1999), leading to a reassessment of manufacturers' liability (*Perez v. Wyeth Laboratories*, 1999).

Quality of Care and E-Health

Consumers continue to increase their reliance on the Web for access to medical information, even though their satisfaction with it may not be high (Landro, 2000), in part, perhaps, because they have relatively low expectations (Harris Interactive, 2000). One initial reaction to the opening of these new channels was frustration over how to manage patients "informed" by indiscriminately selected Web sites. This was followed by concern as to whether to actually recommend some sites (Chin, 2000). Both legal and medical professionals are now detailing their concerns over the quality of online medical interaction (e.g., Medem, 2001a). These concerns over these new channels of communication with patients are not aimed solely at Web advice sites. For example, the AMA (2001d) has called for DTC advertising by pharmaceutical companies ("Direct-to-Consumer Promotion," 1996) to contain disclaimers that physicians might actually recommend other treatments.

Quality of Information

In e-health, even more than in traditional therapist–patient encounters, it is somewhat artificial to draw a distinction between information and advice or treatment. Notwithstanding, the distinction has some merit, because e-health providers tend to emphasize one over the over in defining their business model. Furthermore, when patients allegedly suffer e-health injuries, the characterizations of the services provided likely will have an effect on how courts approach the issues.

The Web is a medium that celebrates new and innovative business models, which more often than not will shun more traditional practices, such as the peer review of medical information. The Web is a medium that prides itself on the very latest information, yet does not have a good track record of reviewing the older data it has published for that data's continued accuracy. Finally, e-health is currently driven not by subscriptions, but instead by advertising or cross-marketing; loyalty, trust, and long-term relationship building are being replaced by "site-stickiness."

Not surprisingly, there have been concerns about the accuracy of online health information. Berland et al. (2001) conducted the most thorough study yet undertaken. Although initially fueling popular press notions of whole-sale inaccuracies (e.g., Hilts, 2001), Berland's quality assessments, particularly for English-language sites, arguably paint a more positive picture than many e-health watchers might have expected. Her most important contribution (and most damaging assessment) is in approaching Web quality assessment as based on a series of factors: search efficiency, topic coverage, and accuracy of information.

As I have pointed out elsewhere (Terry, 1999), malpractice-like actions against Web sites that primarily supply health care information are fraught with technical legal difficulties, including freedom of speech arguments, po-tential statutory immunities (e.g., 47 USC § 230, which arguably provides Internet Service Provider and Web publisher immunity; *Jane Doe One v. Oliver,* 2000), and a sparse history of publishers being held responsible for "advice" or "how-to" books. For some of the same reasons (e.g., the constitutional impli-cations of taking on mere differences of opinion), government agencies tend only to go after the most egregious examples of misleading Web sites (Krebs, 2001). Specifically, they may target sites that promise suspect, fraudulent, or dangerous cures, an issue already raised by Black and Hussain (2000) in the context of Web-purchased hydrazine sulfate being used for cancer therapy. Under the recently announced joint Federal Trade Commission and Food and Drug Administration (FDA) initiative called Operation Cure.All (FTC, 2001; Winter, 2001), considerable federal law enforcement energies are being di-rected against companies marketing fraudulent health products over the Inter-net. Targeted companies are those that market supplements, herbal products, and medical devices that are claimed to treat ailments as diverse as cancer, HIV/AIDS, arthritis, hepatitis, Alzheimer's disease, and diabetes.

Those seeking to make Web-based medical information safe and reliable will have to rely on both market forces strengthening a few well-resourced, trusted sources, and self-regulatory and related technological content solutions. Several highly respected organizations have put forward self-regulatory codes of conduct with accompanying trustmarks, seals, or kitemarks for those who comply. (Health on the Net Foundation, 1997; Hi-Ethics, Inc., 2000; Inter-net Healthcare Coalition, 2000.) A primarily European initiative, MedCertain (www.medcertain.org), is readying a sophisticated system that uses a complex ratings vocabulary and metadata-based content filtering. Simple or sophisti-cated, relying on self-regulation or ratings by third parties, such systems are not without their difficulties (Jadad & Gagliardi, 1998), their critics (Delamothe, 2000), or even their own set of challenging legal issues (Terry, 2000a).

Quality of Care

Notwithstanding the overlap caveat presented earlier, the second broad type of legal issue involves the possible malpractice-like liability of e-therapists. The concerns with online advice or treatment include legal issues such as the existence of a therapist–patient relationship, informed consent to computer-mediated treatment, and digital credentialing. The issues detailed here, however, go to the intrinsic question of the quality of e-therapy.

Anonymized or relatively impersonal communication is viewed as a particular benefit of B2C e-therapy. Yet, this apparently uninhibited, technologically mediated interaction could place the patient in a position to be less honest and more strategic in his or her way of approaching the dialogue. Furthermore, the absence of face-to-face contact removes many of the nonverbal clues from the diagnostic model (Marshall, 2001). At one level, one could ask whether B2C e-therapy is just bad therapy (almost per se malpractice, Almer, 2000; improper diagnosis, Hordern, 2000). At another level, one should question whether very different techniques are required for successful B2C e-therapy, apply selected ones, and study how they influence the quality of care. Therapists considering online interaction with patients also should remember the modern formulation of the *Tarasoff* (*Tarasoff v. Regents*, 1976) duty:

> Since Tarasoff, *a majority of courts that have considered the issue have concluded that the relationship between the psychotherapist and the outpatient constitutes a special relation which imposes upon the psychotherapist an affirmative duty to protect against or control the patient's violent propensities. Recognizing that the duty is imposed by virtue of the relationship, these courts acknowledge that the duty can be imposed not only upon psychiatrists, but also on psychologists, social workers, mental health clinics and other mental health professionals who know, or should have known, of their patient's violent propensities. The courts do not impose any single formulation as to what steps must be taken to alleviate the danger. Depending upon the facts and the allegations of the case, the particular psychotherapist-defendant may or may not be required to perform any number of acts, including prescribing medication, fashioning a program for treatment, using whatever ability he or she has to control access to weapons or to persuade the patient to voluntarily enter a hospital, issuing warnings or notifying the authorities and, if appropriate, initiating involuntary commitment proceedings.* (Estates v. Fairfield Family Counseling Center, 1997)

The reach of this duty is obviously very broad and encompasses most of those likely to be involved in e-therapy. The most sobering feature of the modern psychotherapy duty involves the steps that therapists may have to take to treat patients or to protect third parties. This duty clearly involves steps that would be difficult to take in an exclusively online encounter.

Further issues are raised by the expectations that therapists create with regard to their availability. "24/7" therapy clearly is one of the marketing highpoints of B2C e-therapy. Therapists, however, probably have in mind asynchronous communication and do not intend to have a "live" presence 24 hours per day. During the informed consent process, it should be specified when therapists will not be available, and every Web site should clearly instruct patients what to do in emergency situations.

Similarly, B2C e-therapy scenarios will almost invariably include URLs automatically embedded in e-mail or links from provider Web sites to external content. One question is whether the referrers would face liability for harm caused by the external content if that content had not been explicitly endorsed by particular therapists for particular patients.

A natural reaction of those facing potential liability for e-therapy is to add language to their e-mail communications or Web sites that seeks to reduce legal exposure; however, direct disclaimers of liability for substandard care will have little or no legal effect (*Tunkl v. Regents*, 1963), although in some cases they might chill the litigious urges of e-patients who have not yet sought legal advice. Somewhat more successful will be risk management strategies that seek to reduce litigation (or at least therapists' litigation costs) by inserting what are known as "choice of law" or "forum selection" clauses, aimed at forcing plaintiffs to sue in jurisdictions that are legally or geographically more favorable to defendants (e.g., *Caspi v. Microsoft Network*, 1999), although not all courts accept them (e.g., *Williams v. America Online*, 2001). As a general rule, therapists will have more success with risk management language that explicitly seeks less to exclude litigation, but rather to shape patient expectations and, in particular, to convey the inherent limitations of technologically mediated relationships. Providers should also make available information about to what to do in case of a breakdown in communication (e.g., providing emergency contact information). Inserting such boilerplate language into all e-mail communications is particularly recommended. In practical terms it is more likely to be effective—and less likely to cause the courts to grow weary—than exclusionary language buried on pages deep within Web sites.

Security and Privacy

Many in the health care business regard the HIPAA regulations as an unwelcome and prohibitively expensive piece of overregulation. In fact, those rules, whatever their merits, are merely a means to an end. The "big picture" is so-called "administrative simplification," itself U. S. Department of Health and Human Services (HHS) lingo for reducing administrative and transaction costs that may total as much as $300 billion. The reduction in backend costs associated with billing, reimbursement, insurance claims, and prescription fulfillment is to be achieved by moving the industry to fully interoperable systems for health transactions and promoting efficient health markets. Achieving these goals requires a new, technologically rich architecture for the health system that includes fully digital health records. The key to understanding administrative simplification is the content of the rest of the HIPAA regulatory package. In late 2001, some of these new regulations were not yet available even in draft form (e.g., those specifying codes and data sets for claims attachments, prescription drugs, and national health plan and individual identifiers). Other provisions were available only in draft form (e.g., those providing for national health care provider and employer identifiers).

Security

For this system to be credible and effective, certain patient and system protections are necessary. It is here that HHS has had to enter far more controversial areas, proposing the Security and Electronic Signature Standards ("Notice of a Proposed Rule Making," 1998), and the Standards for Privacy of Individually Identifiable Health Information (PIIHI, 45 CFR §§ 160, 164).

Many of the professional studies on the growing use of communication technologies by physicians have paid particular attention to questions of security (e.g., AMA, 2001b; ISMHO & PSI, 2000a, 2000b; Kane & Sands, 1998; Spielberg, 1998). Data security became a highly visible issue in the mental health arena following a 2000 report that a company that insured almost 2.2 million Californians accidentally sent to the wrong doctors the names of some 12,000 members being treated for depression and anxiety (Wells, 2000).

The draft HIPAA security rules call for both data security and physical security in addition to regulations governing data access and backup, virus control, disaster recovery systems, robust training, and internal policies.

Privacy

Still more controversial have been the PIIHI rules. For U.S. health care providers, the debate has revolved around compliance costs and the extensive civil and criminal sanctions that may be imposed for violations. For others, particularly e-commerce consumers and the trading partners of the United States (particularly the European Union; Directive 95/46/EC, 1995), the controversial issues have been the relatively low level of privacy protection and the inconsistency between different states or industry sectors. According to one EU-commissioned report:

> Internet sites selling products and services to consumers in the United States and Europe fall woefully short of international standards on data protection. Most sites collect personal information but fail to tell consumers how that data will be used, how security is maintained, and what rights consumers have over their own information.
>
> Despite tight European Union (EU) legislation, sites within the EU are no better at providing decent information to their customers than sites based in the US. Indeed some of the best privacy policies are to be found on US sites. . . .
>
> Of sites that collected personal information from their users, health sites were the least likely to have a privacy policy. (Scribbins, 2001, pp. 5, 7)

Almost inevitably, privacy of electronic information became a politically charged issue. Announcing the original PIIHI regulations, former President Clinton stated, "Nothing is more private than someone's medical or psychiatric records" (Department of Health, 2000). Adopting them, albeit with reservations that will lead to their modification, current HHS Secretary Thompson noted, "This town has been debating patient privacy for the better part of a decade, and President Bush believes it is now time to act and protect patients" (Department of Health, 2001).

The hundreds of pages that make up the PIIHI regulations and commentary ("preamble") require that "covered entities" (which include doctors, hospitals, and health—but not life—insurance companies) seek prior consent for any disclosure of "individually identifiable health information." In very general terms, providers must then apply a "minimum necessary" standard to any such disclosure they make. Providers may condition treatment on this consent, but only so far as the disclosure is treatment-centric; no such conditions may be imposed for disclosure of information for, say, marketing use.

The regulations provide for robust (some would say overbroad) exceptions for disclosures to public health and law enforcement entities. Patients are given broad rights to access and to correct their records and can demand an audit of their utilization. True to their HHS source, the privacy rules contain very strong requirements as to compliance policies and systems, including staff training and appointment of a "designated privacy official." Providers are responsible to an extent for unconsented-to disclosures by their "business associates," including law firms and consultants. The regulations provide for stiff civil fines and draconian criminal penalties for knowingly violating patient privacy and will be enforced by the Office for Civil Rights (OCR, 2001). Published guidance from HHS was expected by late 2001, to be followed by modifications to some of the harsher regulatory standards in 2002.

The PIIHI regulations contain Special Rules for Psychotherapy Notes that derogate from the general rules. In particular, psychotherapy notes are "separated from the rest of the individual's medical record" (45 CFR § 164.501), but do not include summaries of the diagnosis or the treatment plan. Special disclosure rules apply (45 CFR § 164.508). Psychotherapy notes are also treated somewhat differently when it comes to rights of patient access [45 CFR § 164.524(a)(1)].

It is important to understand that, uniquely among the HIPAA regulations, the PIIHI rules only partially preempt state law privacy protections. If a state has stronger privacy protections for medical records, they will still be effective after the PIIHI regulations are implemented. Thus, although it is true that the PIIHI rules do not allow for private rights of action by patients, such actions may still be brought against providers on some state theories of liability. Some legislatures are likely to pass state-HIPAA laws that are aimed at specific, identified gaps in the federal regulations (e.g., Texas SB 11).

E-Therapy Promise Versus Legal and Ethical Questions

The adoption of e-health processes and business models will not slow (e.g., PaPeRo, NEC, 2001). Consumer demand—linked to the promise that an infusion of technology will reduce costs and improve quality—will guarantee an increase in B2C e-therapy (Carey, 2000). Indeed:

> E-health has great potential for good. Highly efficient national medical markets, around-the-clock service and the seamless integration of products and services no longer should be the stuff of dreams. The ability to heavily personalize computer-mediated relationships may rehabilitate patient–physician relationships eroded by years of managed care, while the Web's ability to deliver rich information directly to consumers could reverse centuries of damaging informational asymmetry between patient and physician. (Terry, 2001a)

The promises of lower costs and more flexible delivery of services (and not just to rural and other underserved populations) must be seen in the context of the high level of risk associated with unregulated health care delivery. There are also justifiable concerns that the traditional delivery of health care in person will be relegated to the status of a "premium" service, a concept perhaps familiar to psychiatrists who have experienced the restrictions on reimbursement under both managed care and government-funded programs.

Those who do pioneer e-therapy will face considerable legal costs that may be disproportionate to the therapeutic benefits of the new technologies. Indeed, of all medical professionals, psychiatrists are in a particularly difficult situation. Their online activities will not only lead them to compete with other mental health professionals who face far lower entry costs (because psychiatrists attract both the highest level of regulation and the greatest exposure to high damage awards), but also will further blur the scope of practice issues that so trouble the profession.

References

Alabama code § 34-24-74 [Online]. Available: www.legislature.state.al.us/CodeofAlabama/1975/34-24-74.htm

Almer, E. (2000, April 22). Online mental health services: An opportunity, or an alarm? *New York Times* [Online]. Available: www.nytimes.com/library/tech/00/04/biztech/articles/22online.html

AMA survey: Physicians warming up to the Internet. (2001, May 16). *iHealthcareWeekly* [Online]. Available: www.ihealthcareweekly.com/issues/ihcw05162001.html#Headline1178

American Medical Association. (2001a). *Physician licensure: An update of trends* [Online]. Available: www.ama-assn.org/ama/pub/category/2378.html

American Medical Association. (2001b). *Guidelines for physician–patient electronic communications* [Online]. Available: www.ama-assn.org/ama/pub/category/2386.html

American Medical Association. (2001c). *e-Health Initiatives* [Online]. Available: www.ama-assn.org/ama/pub/category/2562.html

American Medical Association. (2001d). *Direct to consumer drug advertising (House of Delegates resolution 503)* [Online]. Available: www.ama-assn.org/ama/pub/category/4940.html

American Psychiatric Association Committee on Telemedical Services. (1998). *American Psychiatric Association resource document on telepsychiatry via videoconferencing* [Online]. Available: www.psych.org/pract_of_psych/tp_paper.cfm

American Psychological Association Ethics Committee. (1997). *Services by telephone, teleconferencing, and Internet* [Online]. Available: www.apa.org/ethics/stmnt01.html

Arizona revised statutes § 36-3601(2) [Online]. Available: www.azleg.state.az.us/ars/36/03601.htm

Arizona revised statutes § 36-3602 [Online]. Available: www.azleg.state.az.us/ars/36/03602.htm

Arkansas code annotated § 17-92-401 [Online]. Available: www.arkleg.state.ar.us/newwebcode/lpext.dll/Infobase/1283f/13983/13e49/13f1d/13f1e

Bates, D. W., & Gawande, A. A. (2000). The impact of the Internet on quality measurement. *Health Affairs, 19*(6), 104–114.

Bates, D. W., Leape, L. L., Cullen, D. J., Laird, N., Petersen, L. A., Teich, J. M., Burdick, E., Hickey, M., Kleefield, S., Shea, B., Vander Vliet, M., & Seger, D. L. (1998). Effect of computerized physician order entry and a team intervention on prevention of serious medication errors. *JAMA, 280,* 1311–1316 [Online]. Available: jama.ama-assn.org/issues/v280n15/abs/joc80319.html

Berland, G. K., Elliott, M. N., Morales, L. S., Algazy, J. I., Kravitz, R. L., Broder, M. S., Kanouse, D. E., Muñoz, J. A., Puyol, J.-A., Lara, M., Watkins, K. E., Yang, H., & McGlynn, E. A. (2001). Health information on the Internet: Accessibility, quality, and readability in English and Spanish. *JAMA, 285,* 2612–2621 [Online]. Available: jama.ama-assn.org/issues/v285n20/abs/joc02274.html

Bienz v. Central Suffolk Hospital. 163 A.D.2d 269 (N.Y. App. Div. 1990).

Black, M., & Hussain, H. (2000). Hydrazine, cancer, the Internet, isoniazid, and the liver. *Annols of Internal Med, 133*(11), 911–913.

Brennan, T. A., Leape, L. L., Laird, N. M., Hebert, L., Localio, A. R., Lawthers, A. G., Newhouse, J. P., Weiler, P. C., & Hiatt, H. H. (1991). Incidence of adverse events and negligence in hospitalized patients. Results of the Harvard Medical Practice Study I. *New England Journal of Medicine, 324,* 370–376.

California business and professions code § 2290.5(a) [Online]. Available: caselaw.lp.findlaw.com/cacodes/bpc/2220-2319.html

Carey, B. (2000, December 11). E-health: Act 2: The scene is changing for online sites as we know them, experts say. What takes their place may be a whole new way of pursuing health care on the Internet. *Los Angeles Times,* p. S1.

Caspi v. Microsoft Network. 323 N.J. Super. 118, 732 A.2d 528 (N.J. Super. Ct. App. Div. 1999) [Online]. Available: media.law.unimelb.edu.au/ehealth/Cases/Caspi_MSN.htm

Chin, T. (2000, October 23/30). Site reading: Physicians grapple with recommending Web sites. *American Medical News* [Online]. Available: www.ama-assn.org/sci-pubs/amnews/pick_00/tesa1023.htm

Code of federal regulations title 45 §160 [Online]. Available: www.access.gpo.gov/nara/cfr/waisidx_01/45cfr160_01.html

Code of federal regulations title 45 §164 [Online]. Available: www.access.gpo.gov/nara/cfr/waisidx_01/45cfr164_01.html

Colorado revised statutes. § 12-36-106(1) [Online]. Available: 64.78.178.125/cgi-dos/statdspp.exe?N&srch=12-36-106

Delamothe, T. (2000). Quality of websites: Kitemarking the west wind. *BMJ, 321,* 843–844 [Online]. Available: www.bmj.com/cgi/content/full/321/7265/843

Department of Health and Human Services. (2000, December 20). *Remarks by the president on medical privacy* [Online]. Available: aspe.hhs.gov/admnsimp/final/whpress2.htm

Department of Health and Human Services. (2001, April 12). *Statement by HHS Secretary Tommy G. Thompson regarding the patient privacy rule* [Online]. Available: http://www.hhs.gov/news/press/2001pres/20010412.html

Directive 95/46/EC of the European Parliament and of the Council of 24 October 1995 on the protection of individuals with regard to the processing of personal data and on the free movement of such data. (1995). Available: europa.eu.int/eur-lex/en/lif/dat/1995/en_395L0046.html

Direct-to-consumer promotion. (1996). 61 Fed. Reg. 24314 [Online]. Available: frwebgate1.access.gpo.gov/cgi-bin/waisgate.cgi?WAISdocID=9574557457+4+0+0&WAISaction=retrieve

Elias, M. (2000, March 7). Online mental-health therapy has issues. *USA Today* [Online]. Available: www.usatoday.com/life/health/mentalh/lhmhe040.htm

Emanuel, E. J., & Dubler, N. N. (1995). Preserving the physician–patient relationship in the era of managed care. *JAMA, 273,* 323–329.

Estates of Morgan v. Fairfield Family Counseling Center. 77 Ohio St.3d 284, 673 N.E.2d 1311 (Ohio 1997) [Online]. Available: www.lawyersweekly.com/ohsup/100018.htm

Eysenbach, G. (2000). Towards ethical guidelines for dealing with unsolicited patient emails and giving teleadvice in the absence of a pre-existing patient–physician relationship—systematic review and expert survey. *Journal of Medical Internet Research, 2*(1). e1. [Online.] Available: www.jmir.org/2000/1/e1

FDA wants to ban personal imports of drugs, except for compassionate uses. (2001, June 8). *BNA Health Care Daily.*

Federal Trade Commission. (2001, June 14). *"Operation Cure.All" wages new battle in ongoing war against Internet health fraud* [Online]. Available: www.ftc.gov/opa/2001/06/cureall.htm

Food and Drug Administration. (2000, February 2). *FDA launches "cyber" letters against potentially illegal, foreign-based online drug sites* [Online]. Available: www.fda.gov/bbs/topics/ANSWERS/ANS01001.html

Frakes v. Cardiology Consultants. 1997 Tenn. App. Lexis 597 (Tenn. Ct. App. 1997) [Online]. Available: media.law.unimelb.edu.au/ehealth/Cases/Frakes.htm

Freudenheim, M. (2001, January 8). Digital doctoring. *New York Times* [Online]. Available: www.nytimes.com/2001/01/08/technology/08HAND.html

Gooden v. Tips. 651 S.W.2d 364 (Tex. Ct. App. 1983) [Online]. Available: media.law.unimelb.edu.au/ehealth/Cases/Gooden.htm

Greene, J. (2001, June 4). "Let the games begin" with interactive CME. *American Medical News* [Online]. Available: www.ama-assn.org/sci-pubs/amnews/pick_01/prl20604.htm

Guidance for industry on consumer-directed broadcast advertisements (1999). 64 Fed. Reg. 43197. [Online.] Available: frwebgate6.access.gpo.gov/cgi-bin/waisgate.cgi?WAISdocID=95754531120+2+0+0&WAISaction=retrieve

Harris Interactive. (2000, October 4). *New survey shows disparity between Web developers and consumers over health Internet* [Online]. Available: www.harrisinteractive.com/news/newscats.asp?NewsID=164

Health on the Net Foundation. (1997). *Health on the Net code of conduct (HONcode) for medical and health websites* [Online]. Available: www.hon.ch/HONcode/Conduct.html

Hi-Ethics, Inc. (2000). *Ethical principles for offering Internet health services to consumers* [Online]. Available: www.hiethics.com/Principles/index.asp

Hilts, P. J. (2001, May 22). Web health info often flawed, new study suggests. *New York Times* [Online]. Available: www.nytimes.com/2001/05/22/health/22CND-NET.html

Hordern, B. B. (2000, July 24). When cybertherapy goes bad. *WebMD* [Online]. Available: my.webmd.com/content/article/1674.50863

Illinois compiled statutes chapter 225 85/16a [Online]. Available: www.legis.state.il.us/ilcs/ch225/ch225act85.htm

Institute of Medicine Committee on Quality of Health Care in America. (2000). *To err is human: Building a safer health system* [Online]. Available: books.nap.edu/books/0309068371/html/index.html

Institute of Medicine Committee on Quality of Health Care in America. (2001). *Crossing the quality chasm: A new health system for the 21st century* [Online]. Available: books.nap.edu/books/0309072808/html/index.html

International Society for Mental Health Online & Psychiatric Society for Informatics. (2000a). *ISMHO/PSI suggested principles of professional ethics for the online provision of mental health services* [Online]. Available: www.ismho.org/suggestions.html

International Society for Mental Health Online & Psychiatric Society for Informatics. (2000b). *ISMHO/PSI suggested principles of professional ethics for the online provision of mental health services* [Online]. Available: www.dr-bob.org/psi/suggestions.3.13.html

Internet Healthcare Coalition. (2000). *eHealth code of ethics* [Online]. Available: www.ihealthcoalition.org/ethics/ehealthcode0524.html

Jadad, A. R., & Gagliardi, A. (1998). Rating health information on the Internet: Navigating to knowledge or to Babel? *JAMA, 279*, 611–614 [Online]. Available: jama.ama-assn.org/issues/v279n8/abs/jrv71042.html

Jane Doe One v. Oliver. 755 A.2d 1000 (Conn. Super. Ct. 2000).

Joy v. Eastern Maine Medical Center. 529 A.2d 1364 (Me. 1987) [Online]. Available: media.law.unimelb.edu.au/ehealth/Cases/Joy_Eastern.htm

Kane, B., & Sands, D. Z. (1998). Guidelines for the clinical use of electronic mail with patients. *Journal of the American Medical Informatics Association, 5*(1), 104–111 [Online]. Available: www.amia.org/pubs/other/email_guidelines.html

Kashishian v. Port. 481 N.W.2d 277, 278 (Wis. 1992) [Online]. Available: media.law.unimelb.edu.au/ehealth/Cases/Kashishian.htm

Krebs, B. (2001, June 11). FTC to take on sites pushing bogus AIDS, cancer cures. *Newsbytes* [Online]. Available: www.newsbytes.com/news/01/166690.html

Kuszler, P. C. (2000). A question of duty: Legal issues resulting from physician response to unsolicited patient e-mail inquiries. *Journal of Medical Internet Research, 2*(3), e17 [Online]. Available: www.jmir.org/2000/3/e17

Landro, L. (2000, December 29). More people are using Internet health sites, but fewer are satisfied. *Wall Street Journal,* p. A9.

MacMillan, R. (2001a, June 6). House panel plans hearing on Net pharmacy risks. *Newsbytes* [Online]. Available: www.newsbytes.com/news/01/166534.html

MacMillan, R. (2001b, June 7). Rep. Stupak to combat Net drug imports—update. *Newsbytes* [Online]. Available: www.newsbytes.com/news/01/166618.html

Marshall, S. (2001, June 10). The therapist is on: Cyber counseling is gaining ground, but critics fear abuse, misdiagnoses. *Washington Post* [Online]. Available: www.washingtonpost.com/wp-dyn/articles/A43307-2001Jun8.html

Matsushita Electric Corporation of America. (2001). *Panasonic telecare solutions* [Online]. Available: www.panasonic.com/telecare

Medem. (2001a). *eRisk guidelines for physician–patient online communications* [Online]. Available: www.medem.com/corporate/corporate_erisk.cfm

Medem. (2001b, April 30). *"Avoid standard un-secure e-mail for online communications with patients,"* says nation's leading medical societies and the AMA, top malpractice carriers and Medem [Online]. Available: www.medem.com/Corporate/press/corporate_medeminthenews_press042.cfm

Microsoft Corporation. (2000, October 3). *.Net for healthcare embraces new Internet standards to revolutionize healthcare* [Online]. Available: www.microsoft.com/presspass/features/2000/Oct00/10-03healthcare.asp

Miller v. Sullivan. 214 A.D.2d 822, 823 (N.Y. App. Div. 1995) [Online]. Available: media.law.unimelb.edu.au/ehealth/Cases/Miller_Sullivan.htm

Montana code annotated § 37-3-341 [Online]. Available: data.opi.state.mt.us/bills/mca/37/3/37-3-341.htm

Montana code annotated § 37-3-342 [Online]. Available: data.opi.state.mt.us/bills/mca/37/3/37-3-342.htm

Montana code annotated § 37-3-343 [Online]. Available: data.opi.state.mt.us/bills/mca/37/3/37-3-343.htm

Mount, C. D., Kelman, C. W., Smith, L. R., & Douglas, R. M. (2000). An integrated electronic health record and information system for Australia? *Medical Journal of Australia, 172,* 25–27 [Online]. Available: www.mja.com.au/public/issues/172_01_030100/mount/mount.html

National Association of Boards of Pharmacy. (1999). *VIPPS* [Online]. Available: www.nabp.net/vipps/intro.asp

NEC Corporation. (2001). *Personal robot PaPeRo* [Online]. Available: www.incx.nec.co.jp/robot/PaPeRo/english/p_index.html

Notice of a proposed rule making for the security and electronic signature standards. (1998) [Online]. Available: aspe.hhs.gov/admnsimp/nprm/seclist.htm

Office for Civil Rights. (2001). *National standards to protect the privacy of personal health information* [Online]. Available: www.hhs.gov/ocr/hipaa

Perez v. Wyeth Laboratories. 734 A.2d 1245, 1263 (N.J. 1999) [Online]. Available: lw.bna.com/lw/19990824/a1698.htm

Posner, E. M. (2000, May 25). *Statement of Ethan M. Posner before the U.S. House of Representatives Committee on Commerce Subcommittee on Oversight and Investigations* [Online]. Available: www.usdoj.gov/criminal/cybercrime/posner.htm

Reason, J. (2000). Human error: Models and management. *BMJ, 320,* 768–770 [Online]. Available: www.bmj.com/cgi/content/full/320/7237/768

Request for comments regarding need for guidance clarifying application of the Internal Revenue Code to use of the Internet by exempt organizations (Announcement 2000–84). (2000, October 16). *Internal Revenue Bulletin, 42,* 385 [Online]. Available: ftp.fedworld.gov/pub/irs-irbs/irb00-42.pdf

Sackett, D. L., Rosenberg, W. M. C., Gray, J. A. M., Haynes, R. B., & Richardson, W. S. (1996). Evidence-based medicine: What it is and what it isn't. *BMJ, 312,* 71–72 [Online]. Available: www.bmj.com/cgi/content/full/312/7023/71

Sands, D. Z., & Bauer, K. (2001, July 2). Build an ethical bridge over the digital divide. *American Medical News* [Online]. Available: www.ama-assn.org/sci-pubs/amnews/pick_01/prca0702.htm

Scribbins, K. (2001, January). *Privacy@net: An international comparative study of consumer privacy on the Internet* [Online]. Available: www.consumersinternational.org/news/pressreleases/privacy250101.html

Silverman, R. D. (2000). Regulating medical practice in the Cyber Age: Issues and challenges for state medical boards. *American Journal of Law & Medicine, 26*(2&3), 255–276.

Spielberg, A. R. (1998). On call and online: Sociohistorical, legal, and ethical implications of e-mail for the patient–physician relationship. *JAMA, 280,* 1353–1359 [Online]. Available: jama.ama-assn.org/issues/v280n15/toc.html

Tapellini, D. (2000, December 7). A wireless doctor is in the house. *Wired* [Online]. Available: www.wired.com/news/technology/0,1282,40560,00.html

Tarasoff v. Regents of the University of California. 17 Cal.3d 425, 551 P.2d 334 (Cal. 1976) [Online]. Available: 129.8.34.16/courses/tarasoff/tarasoff.html

Terry, N. P. (1999). Cyber-malpractice: Legal exposure for cybermedicine. *American Journal of Law & Medicine, 25*(2&3), 327–366 [Online]. Available: papers.ssrn.com/sol3/delivery.cfm/99093014.pdf?abstractid=181976

Terry, N. P. (2000a). Rating the "raters": Legal exposure of trustmark authorities in the context of consumer health informatics. *Journal of Medical Internet Research, 2*(3), e18 [Online]. Available: www.jmir.org/2000/3/e18

Terry, N. P. (2000b). Structural and legal implications of e-health. *Journal of Health Law, 33,* 605–613.

Terry, N. P. (2001a). Access vs quality assurance: The e-health conundrum. *MSJAMA, 285,* 807 [Online]. Available: www.ama-assn.org/sci-pubs/msjama/articles/vol_285/no_5/jms0214014.htm

Terry, N. P. (2001b, June 4). Making a health Web site ethically sound. *American Medical News* [Online]. Available: www.ama-assn.org/sci-pubs/amnews/pick_01/prca0604.htm

Terry, N. P. (2001c). An ehealth diptych: The impact of privacy regulation on medical error and malpractice litigation. *American Journal of Law & Medicine, 27,* 361–419 [Online]. Available: papers.ssrn.com/sol3/delivery.cfm/SSRN_ID286778_code011015140.pdf?abstractid=286778

Texas administrative code §291.34 [Online]. Available: info.sos.state.tx.us/pub/plsql/readtac$ext.TacPage?sl=R&app=9&p_dir=&p_rloc=&p_tloc=&p_ploc=&pg=1&p_tac=&ti=22&pt=15&ch=291&rl=34

Texas administrative code §291.36 [Online]. Available: info.sos.state.tx.us/pub/plsql/readtac$ext.TacPage?sl=R&app=9&p_dir=&p_rloc=&p_tloc=&p_ploc=&pg=1&p_tac=&ti=22&pt=15&ch=291&rl=36

Texas senate bill 11 [Online]. Available: www.capitol.state.tx.us/cgi-bin/db2www/tlo/billhist/Smatrix.d2w/report?LEG=77&SESS=R&CHAMBER=S&BILLTYPE=B&BILLSUFFIX=00011&SORT=Asc

Texas State Board of Medical Examiners. (1999). *Internet prescribing policy* [Online]. Available: www.tsbme.state.tx.us/guidelines/ipp.htm

Top health care information sites in September. (2001, November/December). *Technology in Practice, 2*(9), 9.

Tracy v. Merrell Dow Pharmaceuticals. 569 N.E.2d 875 (Ohio 1991).

Tunkl v. Regents of the University of California. 60 Cal.2d 92, 383 P.2d 441, 32 Cal.Rptr. 33 (Cal. 1963) [Online]. Available: media.law.unimelb.edu.au/ehealth/Cases/Tunkl.htm

U.S. code title 15 §45(a)(1) [Online]. Available: www4.law.cornell.edu/uscode/15/45.html

U.S. code title 42 §1320a-7b [Online]. Available: www4.law.cornell.edu/uscode/42/1320a-7b.html

U.S. code title 42 §1395nn [Online]. Available: www4.law.cornell.edu/uscode/42/1395nn.html

U.S. code title 47 §230 [Online]. Available: www4.law.cornell.edu/uscode/47/230.html

U.S. Department of Justice. (1999, December 9). *Kent Aoki Lee charged by federal grand jury with wire fraud, trademark violations, and selling Viagra over the Internet without a prescription* [Online]. Available: www.cybercrime.gov/kaokilee.htm

VeriSign. (2001, April 25). *American Medical Association partners with VeriSign to launch next generation Internet ID service for health care professionals* [Online]. Available: corporate.verisign.com/news/2001/pr_20010425a.html

Wells, J. (2000, December 30). Wrong MDs got patient records: Psychiatric privacy violated. *San Francisco Chronicle* [Online]. Available: www.sfgate.com/cgi-bin/article.cgi?file=/chronicle/archive/2000/12/30/MNW177137.DTL

West Virginia code §30-3-13 [Online]. Available: www.legis.state.wv.us/scripts/as_web.exe?codesec+D+17689593

White House. (1999, December 28). *Clinton administration unveils new initiative to protect consumers buying prescription drug products over the Internet* [Online]. Available: www.fda.gov/oc/buyonline/onlinesalespr.html

Williams v. America Online. 2001 Mass. Super. Lexis 11 (Mass. Super. Ct. 2001) [Online]. Available: www.socialaw.com/superior/000962.html

Winter, G. (2001, June 15). U.S. crackdown on Net health fraud. *New York Times* [Online]. Available: www.nytimes.com/2001/06/15/technology/15DIET.html

9

My Life as an E-Patient

Martha Ainsworth

IT WAS RAINING THE night I reached the end of my rope. Dark, desolate, dismal—mirroring my mood. Rain, like a heavy curtain, creates a barrier of separation. When it rains, we retreat into the shelter of buildings, shutting doors to protect ourselves from the weather, shutting ourselves away from one another. For some, these shelters may be a warm haven of connectedness, shared with family, colleagues, and friends. But for those who are alone, the curtain of rain magnifies the aloneness, the sense of separation.

As usual, I was alone. In the late afternoon, I had completed one more pre-sentation to one more workshop group that looked like every other workshop group. Temporary relationships, a connection for 3 hours, and then they were gone, home to their families and friends, shutting their doors against the rain, shutting me away, just a passing memory. I was left behind in one more air-port Ramada, one more city like every other city I encountered on that trip. A familiar scenario to be repeated day after day: same script, different people, different city. For several weeks, I could look forward to more of the same.

I needed to talk; there was someone I knew I could call. Even though I knew it was late at night, feeling compelled and reluctant at the same time I dialed anyway, awakening him. Sleepily, he did his best to listen as I struggled to find words to express my desolation. After just a few minutes, he apologized; he just couldn't stay awake. He offered to call the next day. The next day, I would be on a plane, one more plane. Resigned, I hung up the phone. Just another disconnection.

Staring silently out my hotel room window at the rain, I found myself contemplating the state of my life, which was not very good. Too much change, too much loss. A midlife career change that had me grieving the loss of my

194

avowed vocation. The new job, although good, was both stressful and isolating. I had continuing financial struggles. Old emotional wounds forced their way to the surface: a painful divorce, a sense that I could never get close to anyone. As my mind traveled these haunted corridors, I began to feel overwhelmed by grief, loss, and hopelessness.

There is only one thing worse than hopelessness: being alone with it. Turning away from the rain-sodden world in the window, I went to my laptop—and went online.

I went online to cyberspace, to connection—connection with people. It was an association I had learned in 1982, within hours of buying my first computer. I had imagined that "going online" meant nothing more than connecting to another computer to play a game with it. It came as a surprise, and ultimately a delight, to discover there were *people*—hundreds, thousands of real human beings—connecting to each other in cyberspace. I found them in a collectively imagined space called "Participate" in an online world called *The Source*. Before long, I discovered even more cyberspace villages.

Over the next 13 years, I experienced the power of people-to-people cyberspace connections. I made close friends, many of whom I never met in person. I shared my life with them, and they shared theirs with me; we were part of each others' day-to-day lives. Although our bodies were separated by great distances, we were neighbors in the same village, a dynamic community that was always as close to me as my computer.

As the community grew tighter, we began to share more intimate hopes and fears with one another. Soon, we began to form more intentional support groups. Beginning in early 1983, I participated in and led dozens of support groups on a wide variety of topics. A depression support group touched me most. Its members shared deeply with one another and formed an intimate bond that continued for many years. Each person knew that there, in that private cyberspace room, they would find a connection with people who cared. They supported one another through rough times, helped each other cope, bolstered the hope of those whose strength was flagging, and ultimately faced the suicide of one of their own.

Stunned and shaken by that suicide, I realized that as cyberspace continued to expand, similar events would surely follow. I felt compelled to find a way to respond. I immediately set out to learn something about crisis counseling and to adapt it to cyberspace.

People have a tendency to say things online they would never have the courage to say to someone's face (this is known as *disinhibition*). In cyberspace, people share intimate details, hopes, and fears with friends they have never seen—precisely *because* they are unseen. In the privacy of cyberspace, I too could talk more freely about many things. And I witnessed an alarming number of people admit online to despair and suicidal feelings that they would have been embarrassed to acknowledge in person, even to a professional counselor.

As I continued leading support groups, I encountered more and more wounded souls who, freed by the anonymity of online communication, poured forth a seemingly bottomless well of pain. As a compassionate listener, I did the best I could to help, but felt hopelessly inadequate, lacking professional skills and training.

Again and again, my efforts to connect hurting people with psychotherapists were unsuccessful. People seemed to be separated from the help they needed by barriers—misconceptions about psychotherapy, financial and geographic limitations, and most of all, embarrassment. So many people either *could* not or *would* not contact a professional psychotherapist. The intransigence of this gap nagged at me. Psychotherapists know the pain of those who come to them. But the shielding of cyberspace communication was beginning to open a window onto the alarmingly huge population of walking wounded who had never made it to psychotherapists' offices.

Often, I wished that all those people who found it so much easier to speak their innermost thoughts online could have had someone to listen who could actually have helped. I prayed for the day when professional psychotherapists would cross the barrier, venture into cyberspace, and take a step closer to those isolated, hurting people who could not come to them.

I had to wait 13 years.

By 1995, the old online services were giving way to e-mail and the Web. And now I was myself one of those wounded souls, looking for someone who could hear my pain, accept me, care both about me and for me. I was looking for this person in the middle of the night, and I was not looking for an office. I wanted to find this person in cyberspace, where I knew it would be safe to talk.

With the help of a search engine, I began to find Web pages on which psychotherapists advertised their office practices. No, I thought to myself, that's not what I need. I want to work with someone *here*, wherever "here" happened to be for me from one day to the next. I needed to dig deeper.

I found the page of a psychotherapist who offered to respond to one question for a small fee, sort of a psychological Ann Landers. But nowhere on the Web site did the therapist reveal his or her name or location. That made me very uneasy. How could I know for sure that this was really a competent professional?

Another site seemed promising, but the intake form, which was not secure, demanded my name, credit card number, street address, and phone number, which I was not prepared to surrender to a total stranger. I continued clicking.

I came across a site where, again, psychotherapists offered to answer questions for a small fee. They did give their names and professional qualifications, so I felt more reassured. I clicked to the submission form and began trying to frame my question. After half an hour, I gave up. I didn't have a "question." I wasn't looking for an "answer." I was looking for a person, a relationship. One e-mail was not going to be enough. I kept searching.

Finally, 2 hours later, I clicked on a page that began:

WELCOME TO THE MENTAL HEALTH CYBER-CLINIC

Within a paragraph or two, I could see that this place was different. I saw the words "ongoing helping dialogue," and my heart leapt. Was this someone who would be there for me, who would be willing to stick with me for awhile?

The therapist had written several pages describing the e-therapy helping process. His tone was informal, but professional. The language was first–second person, "I" and "you"; reading his words, I seemed to be in a conversation with him. He quite obviously was an extremely competent psychotherapist who also understood the Internet. He wrote insightfully about e-mail and online communication. From his writing style, I could see that he knew how to communicate in writing; his gentle compassion shone through his words. Best of all, he spoke of forming a *relationship*. As I read, I began to feel that he would be willing and able to listen to me.

As he described what he could offer, he was thorough and upfront about the limitations and risks, as well as the possibilities, of working together online. It made me feel that he was responsible, that he cared about my welfare, that he would not try to "sell" me something. He was not pushing a book or massaging his ego by promoting his own theory of psychotherapy. He wasn't talking about himself, he was talking about me . . . about us. He was winning my trust before he ever knew of my existence.

I knew enough about cyberspace to be cautious. Things are not always as they seem. But the therapist provided his résumé, complete with license number, office address, and telephone number. My sense of trust began to take hold.

My decision to reach out to him was almost not of my own volition. The pain in my soul was overflowing, and this therapist seemed to have his arms open, waiting to take it from me. I quickly clicked through to the short intake form.

I started to fill out the form . . . then hesitated. I was about to reveal intimate details about myself to a total stranger. Inside, I felt conflicted. I wanted desperately to connect to this person. Yet at the same time, I was wary and wanted to protect myself. I scanned the form and saw that he did not ask for my name or any other identifying information beyond my e-mail address. Something inside me relaxed. I could reveal to him only as much as I felt comfortable revealing. There was nothing intrusive here; only hospitality and an invitation to talk. He was not demanding anything, only accepting whatever I cared to share. I felt I had some control. I completed the form and sent it off.

We had already had our first session, and the therapist didn't even know it yet.

The next day, my attitude toward physical aloneness had completely reversed. On the plane, I fidgeted, impatient to be alone in my hotel room. I wanted to check my e-mail. I *really* wanted to check my e-mail. The flight seemed endless. My thoughts kept going to the "Mental Health Cyber-Clinic." Was this therapist real? Would he care about me? Would he really be there? Maybe there would be no response at all. Maybe it would be a disappointment. Finally, I reached the hotel and checked in. I hurried to the room, flung the suitcase on the bed, and went directly to the desk and phone. My hands were trembling as I connected the laptop to the phone line. Would I get a response to the cry of pain I had sent off into cyberspace? Would it be human, or would it be a form letter? Could I make a connection with a person who cared?

My heart stopped as my e-mail inbox came up. Yes! There it was:

Subject: 2 e-mails from the cyber-clinic

With some trepidation, I opened the e-mail. I remember scanning the text quickly. Two sentences seemed to leap from the page:

I am here for you and will try only to help.
I am very concerned about you.

With those two sentences, he completed the circle. He *had* heard me and grasped my pain; he had responded with caring. My human need cried out, and his human compassion responded. It was *connection*. Physically, we were separated by five states; but psychically, we were more connected than if we had been in the same room. In that moment, a relationship came into being that grew into one of the most profound I have ever known.

I read the remainder of the e-mail more carefully. He established the therapeutic frame, explaining ground rules and procedures, and offered a few gently probing questions based on the form I had completed, about my family, my history, and so on, to help me start telling my story. "Mostly questions to start with," he said, "as I need to know you better, and you need to know me too." The e-mail ended:

> *Let's try to keep the dialogue going so that not too much time elapses between our e-mails.*
> *Is telephone therapy a possibility?*
> *Can I have at least a first name?*
> *I hope to hear from you soon.*

I felt an enormous sense of relief. Not only was he caring and willing to help, but the fact that we were meeting through the anonymity shield of cyberspace made me feel free to tell him everything. I started composing my response right away. I wrote, and wrote, and wrote some more, ending with:

> Have I scared you off yet?
> I find myself stranded and feeling extremely reluctant about entering into a therapy relationship. I am feeling timid about you. The thought of going through that is overwhelming right now. I am of uncertain hope about whether it can be helpful. And the recent feelings I have been having is stuff I never could talk about to anyone. I write better than I talk. The anonymity of online communication, etc., etc. You know all that. I do not talk well at all.
> My name is Martha.
> I'm not quite ready for the telephone. I'm really not good at talking on the phone, it makes me very self-conscious. Can we just keep writing?
> I am scheduled to be traveling for the next several weeks. I have a laptop that I take with me. I envision being in my hotel room at night, alone and isolated, far from home. I envision e-mail as a potential lifeline.

Once again I hit the *send* button, as I had done 24 hours before. But now it was a very different experience. No longer was I sending my innermost thoughts into a black hole in cyberspace. I felt a living strand of connection between myself and another human being who, although he was several states away, was beginning to create a presence as close as my own thoughts. Because I had no physical manifestation to which I could relate, he existed inside my own head, to be carried around with me throughout the day.

Day by day, he drew me out, helping me talk about the pain. Within a few days, I had told him my whole life story (or so I thought). Late at night, when I felt most alone, I sat down at the computer to write. Sometimes, I wrote again early in the morning. During the day, he always responded within a few hours. It became apparent that just as I held him in my mind, the same was true for him; he held me in his thoughts. I felt totally connected to him—to this caring presence I had never seen in person.

His questions gradually got deeper and more difficult, as did my responses. Little by little, as my trust deepened, I yielded up more information about myself—the city and state where I lived, my last name. I still didn't give up my telephone number. I felt I needed that distance to enable me to continue talking. He was gentle but persistent.

Perhaps a short-term goal should be to say hello on the phone even for a minute.

No, I'm really resistant about talking on the phone. I have a sort of phone phobia. Talking is really hard for me. Everyone says that I am a very quiet person. What's going on in my mind is not quiet, but getting it from my brain out of my mouth is exceedingly difficult, for a whole variety of historical reasons. I always found it very tough to talk on the phone. So, maybe sometime we will talk on the phone, but not yet. The thought scares me a lot.

As the weeks went on, the closeness deepened. As is often the case in cyberspace relationships, we began to fantasize about what it would be like to meet for a therapy session in person.

I feel a desire to sit down in my office with you, and I recognize that this is not possible. I feel a need to "embrace" you (figuratively) and stand with you through all your struggles.

I feel that too. I found myself looking at a map to find out how long it takes to drive to your city. But the thing is, there are things I can talk about in this way that I can't approach face to face. What I write to you is much more "inner" than what I would probably tell you in person. So let's continue trailblazing here in e-mail.

My e-therapist had two outstanding qualities that never ceased to amaze me: intuition and strength. To this day, I am not sure how he did it, but he was nearly always able to sense my moods accurately, just from my writing. I went through a dizzying range of emotions: depression, playfulness, rage, despair, terror. He always knew.

This day started bad and got worse. The constant ache at the center of my soul. Now it feels like a searing pain. I fear I will always feel this way. I am so tired . . . If you are the one who is so hopeful then give me a reason to keep this up, to keep corresponding with you. Why I am doing this? Why am I trying at all?

Martha,
I feel your pain and anger to the extent possible over our connection. You know I am here. I don't want to be completely quiet because I don't want you to think I am stuck. So what

to do? I am going to trust your inner strength and God's will that there is a way out of this mess for you. I will stand by your side as you travel that way, respecting your silence as needed.

No! Now I *am* angry. I *don't* want you to "respect" my silence, dammit, I want you to break into it. And no, *I* don't know what that means, I need *you* to know. You say you will "stand by"?? I don't know what I want from you, but please don't abandon me here, don't stand by and watch.
You said, "I don't want to be completely quiet because I don't want you to think I am stuck. So what to do?"
I don't know, but figure it out, okay?

I'm sorry I yelled at you earlier. I hope you are not angry at me. The last thing I need right now is to be abandoned. I imagine that you are having second thoughts about having gotten involved with me.

Martha,
Please know and trust that I am not angry with you.
It is noteworthy, the quickness with which you seemed to assume I would somehow reject you.
I will not deny that I wish I could do more for you and am thus a little frustrated, but the thought of bailing out never crossed my mind. We are in the present, not your past.

The strength of our therapeutic frame was unwavering. No matter what I threw at him, he was rock solid, firmly optimistic, gentle, and loving. I told him horrible things from the depths of my depression, and he was not horrified; he accepted them calmly. I raged, and he accepted it calmly. I transferred onto him the abandonment, abuse, neglect, and incomprehension I had suffered from others. Knowing it for what it was, he accepted it calmly and responded with caring and warmth. No matter how hard I slammed into the frame, it was always strong enough to hold me. Our relationship was a well of caring that to this day has never run dry.

Dear Martha,
You have been on my mind since yesterday. I am wondering, how are you doing today? Do you have any periods of respite from your feelings? What are your thoughts like at the best times? The worst?

In the moment, when you asked, "how are you feeling today?" I honestly couldn't answer because on the spot in that moment I truly didn't know. It took a long time, thinking about it, before I could say, yes, I feel . . . like crying. Sad. Hopeless. So I suppose that asynchronous therapy works for me in one sense, because my feelings are usually asynchronous to the event with which they're supposed to be associated. E-mail gives me a chance to catch up.

What I am feeling is loss, or maybe it's just an aching loneliness. Writing to you opened a wound. As if your kindness made me realize fully how bad I feel. The fact that you asked—that one person on this planet wants to know how I feel—took a cork off a bottle somewhere inside, and I've spent the last couple of hours crying. My feelings were frozen, and you made them melt, and now instead of ice I have this lake of emotions filling up again.

My feelings seem toxic. It's like a lake that keeps filling, threatening to overflow. There is no way to drain the lake. The toxic thoughts and feelings are trapped and have no outlet, because no one really wants to hear me talk about it. Except you.

The metaphor of the lake is interesting—let's work with that. First let's stem the springs that feed the lake from the inside. Then let's spill some of the toxic "water" off the top, so that the lake's level is well below the overflow mark. You must be able to talk about your life in your protected space, and you need to not be alone there.

You know, as I sit here and think about you, Martha, I find myself wanting to go into that lake with you, swim around awhile, check out all its features, see how clean the water is, or isn't, and then maybe call the Army Corps of Engineers and tell them the lake is a flood hazard, so we need to build some drainage. Real good drainage, bomb proof and all that. Let the water drain into the vastness of God's oceans which can easily absorb the water. Then in the dry land which remains plant flowers and fruit trees. They would grow slowly in the lush soil, but fully. Bearing beautiful blossoms and petals each year, forever.

Martha, you are a kind person, whose woundedness helps her to feel compassion for others and whose life work is meaningful. Write with you tomorrow.

Eventually, we did speak on the phone. Nine months later, we met in person, and have done so perhaps a half-dozen times in 5 years. Strangely, when I finally did sit down with him in his therapy office, it wasn't the same. He was just as caring, just as warm, just as insightful. But because he was there in person, I found that there were things I could not say. And predictably, when I got home from that visit, all the things I had been unable to say in person came out in e-mail.

Our correspondence continued for over 2 years. My e-therapist was faithful, and his caring for me has never wavered. I was challenged, comforted, and empowered. The experience was profoundly healing, and my life changed for the better.

I now have a wonderful, deep, trusting relationship with another very gifted, loving therapist, with whom I meet in the traditional way, in an office for weekly sessions. But as close as I am to him, there are still things I cannot say when I am in his presence. When I have something very difficult to talk about, I return to the private, shielded, nonvisual connection of e-mail.

ABCs of Internet Therapy: Metanoia.org

Metanoia: Greek word meaning "a change of mind"

When I had been working with my e-therapist for a few months, I recognized the power of our relationship and how much it was helping me. I thought about all those wounded people I had come to know in online support groups. I realized that they and others might also find help working with a therapist online. I decided to publish a list of e-therapists to make it easier for other people in pain to find help, as I had done.

That first night I had searched the Internet for a therapist, I had found 12 Web sites where psychotherapists offered to interact with people online. Six months later, in the spring of 1996, there were about 50. Obviously, I was not the only one finding value in this medium.

As I began to compile the list, visiting all 50 sites, I had a strong reaction to what I was seeing. The differences in e-therapy Web sites were extreme. Some were very professional, others quite amateurish. On some, I found things that alarmed me as a consumer advocate: therapists who did not disclose their credentials, a few who did not even reveal their names. How could we, as consumers, judge whether they were competent to help us? On several sites, therapists were asking e-patients to send credit card numbers by e-mail, potentially very risky. Some openly admitted that the e-patient's messages might be received by someone other than the therapist. And on one or two sites, I never did receive a response to my e-mail. This is comparable to a therapist who does not bother to pick up messages from his or her answering machine.

It was apparent that some education was needed. There were trust issues in both directions. E-therapists, out of their own wariness as well as professional responsibility, were demanding information from e-patients, but they were not reciprocating. Many e-therapists were not paying attention to consumer confidence issues; apparently they did not realize the unconscious effect this might have on therapeutic communication with e-patients. Trust is an essential ingredient in a therapy relationship. I doubt the e-therapists were violating this trust intentionally; they were simply unaware.

It was even more apparent to me that consumers of online therapy needed education, to be more assured of getting appropriate help. When we are in pain, we tend to be indiscriminate; we reach for the first seemingly caring person we find. Unfortunately, if that first relationship goes wrong, many people may never attempt it again, choosing continued suffering over the risk of another failure in therapy. Some of the sites I found alarmed me—some self-styled "counselors" were nothing more than advice columnists with no mental health credentials at all. I felt something needed to be said.

During my work with online support groups, I had written extensively about how to choose a competent psychotherapist. I believed very strongly that patients should be proactive and take responsibility for their choice of psychotherapist. The vast majority of psychotherapists and counselors were competent, responsible professionals. But, unfortunately, a number of psychotherapists out there were incompetent, some dangerously so. Consumers must know what they may expect from a psychotherapist so that they can recognize the difference between a competent therapist and one who is not. Abandoning my responsibility to other e-therapy patients would allow less-than-reputable counselors to take advantage of the vulnerability of people in pain.

With all this in mind, I created "ABCs of Internet Therapy" (www. metanoia.org) in the spring of 1996. I had two missions:

1. To create and maintain a directory of professional psychotherapists who worked with people via the Internet.
2. To educate consumers about e-therapy, enabling them to make responsible choices and to be more ensured of getting appropriate help.

There is nearly universal agreement that the helping relationships offered by professional psychotherapists via the Internet are not "psychotherapy," and there is no danger that e-therapy will ever replace traditional psychotherapy. However, it is quite clear that there is still enormous helping potential when therapists talk with people on the Internet. Emotional support, interactive journaling, psychoeducation, customized information, and advice are all types of helping that, although they fall short of "psychotherapy," are effective ways of caring. Perhaps most important, these Internet interactions have made help available to people who had no other access to psychotherapy.

What follows here is material adapted from "ABCs of Internet Therapy". I first offer a brief history and survey of the e-therapy field as it existed in the year 2002 (when I wrote this chapter). Following that, I have some advice for e-patients and other advice for e-therapists. I close with some philosophical observations.

Surveying the E-Therapy Field

Almost as soon as the Internet was invented, its potential for psychotherapeutic communication was apparent. One of the first demonstrations of the Internet was a simulated psychotherapy session between computers at Stanford and UCLA during the International Conference on Computer Communication in October 1972.

Online self-help support groups were the precursor to e-therapy; the enduring success of these groups has firmly established the potential of computer-mediated communication to enable discussion of sensitive personal issues. Local computer bulletin board systems began to develop not long after the introduction of the first personal computers in 1976; it is not unreasonable to assume that small, informal support groups gathered on some of them. Beginning in 1979, when the first national online services (The Source and Compuserve) allowed nationwide online communication for personal computer users, it was not long until formally organized online support groups became popular. I personally organized such groups as early as 1982.

It is not possible to know precisely when mental health professionals began interacting with patients online. As long as psychotherapists have participated in online activities and have been known to be psychotherapists, they have probably received requests for help, and some have probably responded. Thus, the earliest history of e-therapy is lost in confidential obscurity.

The earliest known organized service to provide mental health advice online was "Ask Uncle Ezra" (cuinfo.cornell.edu/Dialogs/EZRA), a free service offered to students of Cornell University in Ithaca, NY. "Ask Uncle Ezra" (named for Ezra Cornell, the university's founder) was initiated by Jerry Feist (at that time Director of Psychological Services) and Steve Worona, and has been in continuous operation since September 1986.

Ivan Goldberg, M.D., began fielding questions online about the medical treatment of depression at least as early as 1993. He did not solicit questions on his own popular Web site, "Depression Central" (www.psycom.net/depression.central.html), but generously served as unofficial advisor to the online depression support group "Walkers in Darkness," responding to inquiries about medications in an "educational" capacity. John Grohol, Psy.D., has offered free mental health advice in a popular weekly public chat (psych-central.com/chats.htm) since 1995.

Fee-based mental health services began to be offered to the public on the Internet in mid-1995. Most were of the "mental health advice" type, offering to answer one question for a small fee. The earliest such practitioner was Leonard Holmes, Ph.D., who offered "Shareware Psychological Consultation" (www.leonardholmes.com), answering questions on a "pay if it helps" basis. Holmes reported that as soon as he set up a Web site advertising his practice, he began to receive e-mail from people asking for help; it was apparent that people were ready to reach out to psychotherapists via the Internet (personal communication, November, 2000). "Help Net" and "Shrink Link" were two other fee-based mental health advice Web sites available in the fall of 1995 (neither is still online).

David Sommers, Ph.D., may be considered the primary pioneer of e-therapy. He was the first to establish a fee-based Internet service that attempted to do more than answer a single question; he sought to establish longer-term, ongoing helping relationships, communicating only via the Internet. From 1995 through 1998, Sommers worked with over 300 persons in his online practice, spanning the globe from the Arctic Circle to Kuwait. Sommers employed several consumer-level Internet technologies for e-therapy—primarily e-mail with encryption, but also real-time chat and videoconferencing.

Ed Needham, M.S., established his "Cyberpsych" Internet Relay Chat service (www.win.net/cyberpsych) in August 1995, and was the first to focus exclusively on e-therapy interaction via real-time chat. He worked with 44 persons from 1995 to 1998. Other early explorers of ongoing e-therapy included the Pink Practice, in London (www.pinkpractice.co.uk).

The development of hospital- and clinic-based telemedicine—the use of sophisticated videoconferencing hookups to allow physicians to work with patients in remote locations—has been well documented elsewhere.

Although they are not professional psychotherapists, no survey of Internet helping relationships would be complete without mention of the Samaritans (www.samaritans.org.uk). These trained volunteer crisis counselors have answered e-mail from despairing and suicidal persons daily since 1994, anonymously and without charge. Their lifesaving work has been of immeasurable value. In 1999 alone, Samaritan volunteers responded to e-mail from 25,000 persons. Originally handled by one Samaritan branch in Gloucester, U.K., e-mail services are now available at 21 branches, including Hong Kong and Perth.

In the fall of 1995, when I did my own search, I found 12 e-therapists practicing on the Internet. My database has now grown to include over 300 private-practice Web sites where e-therapists offer services and the newer "e-clinics," which represent, collectively, nearly 500 more e-therapists. And the number is growing.

At the beginning of the 21st century, interaction between mental health professionals and consumers on the Internet may be divided into four types. Two types of interaction take place entirely via the Internet, whereas the others combine Internet communication with in-person treatment:

- *E-therapy:* Psychotherapists form ongoing helping relationships that take place solely via Internet communication. This term was first coined by John Grohol, Psy. D.
- *Mental health advice:* Psychotherapists respond to one question in depth, again with communication taking place solely via the Internet.
- *Adjunct services:* Psychotherapists use Internet communication to supplement traditional, in-person treatment.
- *Behavioral telehealth and telepsychiatry:* Mental health professionals (typically psychiatrists) use sophisticated videoconferencing systems to work with patients in remote locations as an extension of traditional clinic or hospital care.

These four types of interaction are very different, although each uses telecommunication in some way. A separate volume could be written about each. Although all have great promise, my primary focus has been on the field of e-therapy. I believe that e-therapy has the most potential to reach the people who particularly concern me: troubled and despairing people for whom traditional mental health treatment is inaccessible.

It is worth noting that adjunct services, although not often publicized, are used increasingly by many psychotherapists in the same way as telephone conversations, to communicate with patients between sessions or to keep in touch with patients who have moved or are traveling. As mental health professionals become more accustomed to using the Internet and discover the disinhibiting effect of online communication, they are beginning to take advantage of it and to incorporate it into their relationships with the patients they see in person.

E-therapists are exploring all modes of Internet communication for their work with e-patients. Services are currently available using e-mail (regular or encrypted), real-time chat, secure Web-based messaging, videoconferencing, and voice-over-Internet Protocol (Internet phone). Many e-therapists offer more than one of these modes, giving the e-patient a choice based on preference and available technology. As broadband Internet connections become available to more consumers, videoconferencing and Internet phone are increasingly available. Even so, many consumers continue to prefer the nonvisual, nonvoice, low-tech environment of e-mail and chat, finding it easier to communicate about sensitive issues without visual or voice connection.

The advent of large, commercial e-clinics marked a significant development in e-therapy. These business ventures seek to offer an improved environment for e-therapy by offering resources most independent e-therapists cannot afford: the most robust online security possible, credit card billing services and other practice management tools, thorough screening of clinicians, and active marketing. Therapists may join these e-clinics for a modest monthly fee and are offered a boilerplate Web page through which they may conduct their own e-therapy practice. Consumers who visit the sites are offered a list of e-therapists from whom to choose, all of whom have been carefully screened to ensure that they are qualified professionals. Other features include the ability to select a therapist according to various criteria, access to self-help information, and support groups for members. "HelpHorizons.com" (www.helphorizons.com) and "Find-A-Therapist" (e-therapyhelper.com) are examples of e-clinics.

A milestone in the development of e-therapy was the formation of the International Society for Mental Health Online (ISMHO, www.ismho.org). ISMHO is a nonprofit society formed by myself and others in 1997 to promote the understanding, use, and development of online communication, information, and technology for the international mental health community. It has become the unofficial professional organization for e-therapists, providing peer support and insightful discussion as mental health professionals seek responsible ways to use the Internet to provide mental health help. ISMHO provides a public discussion forum (accessible from the Web site) in addition to a members-only area. Perhaps most important, it sponsors a clinical case study group that provides valuable insights into new clinical issues and intervention formats developing on the Internet.

Providing support for consumers, Metanoia.org addresses the issues that are important for prospective e-patients to consider. I educate consumers about the opportunities and dangers presented by working with a therapist online, including ethics, privacy, and legal issues.

Over the course of 4 years, I have offered on my site a consumer satisfaction survey, which has yielded some interesting information. In May 1999, out of 619 total responses, 452 respondents (73%) had tried e-therapy. Of those, 416 (92%) said that it had helped them, and 307 (68%) said that they had never been in therapy before contacting a therapist via the Internet.

The data seem to suggest that many of those who are drawn to contact a therapist on the Internet do so because, for them, traditional psychotherapy is not accessible. The most common reason for inaccessibility is stigma; many people are too embarrassed to make in-person contact with a psychotherapist. *Mental Health: A Report of the Surgeon General* (U.S. Department of Health and Human Services, 1999) revealed that nearly two-thirds of people who need mental health care never get it, and cited stigma as a primary reason.

It is not news that traditional mental health care serves only a fraction of the population who need it. To many people, the Internet feels more private, and this perceived privacy helps them get past the barrier of stigma to seek help through e-therapy. Interestingly, in my survey, of the 307 persons for whom e-therapy was their first contact with a therapist, 197 (64%) eventually moved on to consult a therapist in person.

It would appear that, as I had hoped, the Internet is providing a bridge across one of the barriers that keeps people from getting the help they need. As psychotherapists have ventured into this cyberspace sanctuary—where people find it easier to speak their innermost thoughts—more and more people who would not otherwise have been helped are finding a path to healing.

Guidance for E-Patients

I would like to address a few words to readers who may be considering consulting a psychotherapist via the Internet. Before you do, there are some things you must consider.

E-therapy may be a viable alternative source of help when traditional psychotherapy is not accessible. It's effective. It's private. It's conducted by skilled, qualified, ethical professionals. And for some people, it's the only way they can get help from a professional therapist.

E-therapy will never replace traditional psychotherapy. Working with a therapist in person is still better. But many people cannot or will not see a therapist in person. E-therapy is a form of counseling that, although it falls short of full-fledged psychotherapy, is still a very effective way of being helped.

If you are someone who is troubled and seeking help, perhaps you are wondering: How can e-therapy help?

Things happen in life that are normal—we all face them—but are difficult. A big change in your life... loss of a job, or a home, or an important relationship... emotions and feelings that seem overwhelming... challenges of parenting and family life... troubling relationships... difficulties at work.

When these things happen to you, it doesn't mean there is anything wrong with you; it doesn't mean you are "mentally ill." These things happen to everybody. Why would you want to go through them alone?

A therapist is trained to help you cope with these things, so you can get through them and feel happier. Psychotherapists can be there for you. Now, some of them are there for you on the Internet.

E-therapy is not appropriate for everyone. And, as with any new frontier, there are some issues you should consider before venturing forth. But even so, there is a basic truth: Every day, responsible, competent, ethical mental health professionals are forming effective helping relationships via the Internet—relationships that help and heal.

Ask yourself the following questions before you consult an e-therapist.

Is E-Therapy Right for You?

- It's a good option for many people, but not everyone. The biggest risk of e-therapy is that someone will use it who shouldn't. E-therapists do their best to make sure you are an appropriate candidate for e-therapy before starting to work with you, but you share responsibility for this decision.
- E-therapy is not recommended for people who are in the midst of a serious crisis. There are other, better ways to get immediate crisis help.
- E-therapy is still in a formative stage. You must understand and be comfortable with the risks as well as the advantages. Many people are being helped, but you need to know what the issues are.
- If you're going to work with a therapist by e-mail or chat, you must be comfortable writing expressively, informally, and in some detail. If you don't like writing, look for a therapist who is available by videoconferencing or Internet phone.
- You must be willing to reveal yourself to the therapist. If you conceal important feelings or information about yourself, you will only be hurting yourself (and wasting your money). Because the therapist won't have all the usual visual clues, you must work a little harder.
- If your situation is very complex or you have some really tough problems, e-therapy may be a short-term solution at best. If the therapist feels you need more help than he or she can give you, the therapist will tell you so and refer you to another source of help. For some people, a few sessions with a therapist online are enough; but if it's appropriate, and if it's possible, most e-therapists will like for you to see a therapist in person.

Who Is the Therapist?

Make sure the therapist is qualified to help you. Never initiate contact with a therapist unless you verify his or her credentials or check that they have been verified by a neutral third party. Get real-world contact information to use in case of a computer problem. A responsible therapist will gladly give his or her full name, credentials, location, and office telephone number.

What Will the Therapist Provide, and How Much Will It Cost?

Make sure that you'll actually get a personal reply, and ask how long it will take. Find out in advance how much the therapist charges and what forms of payment the therapist accepts.

Will Your Privacy Be Protected?

- If online security concerns you, use encrypted e-mail. Secure, web-based communication systems are also available that do not store your messages on your own computer and thus keep your communications safer from prying eyes.
- Never leave your computer unattended while it is running—especially while it is connected to the Internet and other people are around. If you walk away, start a password-protected screen saver or security program.
- Make sure other persons cannot sit down at your computer and send or receive e-mail. Do not store your e-mail password in your e-mail program; set it up so that you must type your password every time to send or receive e-mail.
- If you share your computer with anyone else (including family members), password-protect your files.
- For passwords, select apparently meaningless strings of characters, not words. Include punctuation if possible.
- Doublecheck every e-mail before sending it to be sure it is correctly addressed.
- If you print e-mail on paper, safeguard the paper.
- If you use a laptop or handheld computer, be very careful to prevent its theft.
- Don't e-mail your therapist from work; your employer has a legal right to read any e-mail on your computer there.

Guidance for E-Therapists

I also have some comments to address to psychotherapists who may be considering providing services via the Internet.

For the protection of consumers, certain information should be provided on an e-therapy site. If you plan to offer e-therapy, please be sure that prospective e-patients can access all of the following information *before* deciding whether to pay for your services.

Information About You

Mutual trust is essential in the online relationship between e-therapist and e-patient. I say "mutual" because it goes both ways: E-patients want assurance that you are a bonafide therapist, and you want assurance that patients are legitimate. Unfortunately, there are some frauds out there in cyberspace. Prospective e-patients rely on you to tell them who you really are and whether you really are a qualified therapist. It is essential that you put their minds at ease by providing them with enough information to verify your credentials independently and to contact you offline, if necessary. You must provide:

- Your real name.
- Your physical location (at minimum, the state or province and the country where you practice; preferably also the city, although not necessarily your street address).
- Your office telephone number.
- Your discipline (i.e., psychologist, marriage and family counselor, social worker, pastoral counselor, etc.).
- Your credentials (i.e., certification, license, registration, etc.), with enough details to allow e-patients to contact the credentialing organizations to verify your credentials independently.

Information About Your Services

The only complaints I've ever received from e-patients were about money. If the e-therapists had been upfront about the cost, the misunderstandings would have been avoided. Prospective e-patients need to know how much money they will spend and what they may expect to receive for it:

- You must tell them how much you charge (e.g., "US$20.00 for each e-mail I write").
- If you plan to charge "per minute" for answering e-mail, state upfront what the total cost is likely to be, and set a "cap" or maximum amount you will charge per e-mail. I've received more than one consumer complaint about unexpectedly large bills. Be clear about the cost.
- Explain the payment options you offer (i.e., check, money order, credit card, electronic check, charge to phone bill, PayPal, etc.).

- If you accept credit cards, you must allow payment through a secure server or by telephone or fax. There is *no excuse* for requiring e-patients to send credit card information by e-mail or through a nonsecure Web form. There are low-cost methods of accepting credit card payments online.

Be conscious of the nervousness prospective e-patients feel as they try to decide whether or not to enter into a relationship with you. It's important for you to reassure them and to build a therapeutic frame, just as you would with patients in person.

State on your site whether e-patients will receive personal, private responses from you and, if so, when they may expect your responses (i.e., within 24 hours, 48 hours, 3 weeks, etc.). Explain how you will communicate (i.e., by e-mail, live chat, videoconferencing, Web-based messaging, Internet phone, etc.). State whether you offer encryption.

If more than one e-therapist offers services on your site, it is important for prospective e-patients to be able to choose in advance which e-therapists they will work with.

Finally, inform prospective e-patients about the limitations of e-therapy (e.g., what problems you consider to require treatment in person), and the limits to confidentiality, both in general (e.g., when involving child abuse) and online (e.g., due to hackers).

If you are beginning to explore e-therapy, I highly recommend that you join the International Society for Mental Health Online (www.ismho.org). This organization provides the best available peer support for e-therapists, and intelligent, open discussion of the issues.

Good luck, and when you get a site going, let me know through Metanoia.org.

E-Therapy Ethics: A Consumer's Opinion

Finally, I would like to offer my own opinion with regard to e-therapy ethics. I am a consumer and consumer advocate who has observed this field closely since the fall of 1995. Do I advocate e-therapy? My only desire is for all humans in emotional difficulty to get compassionate, professional help. When e-therapy can accomplish that, I will advocate it. And when there is danger of harm, I will warn against it.

Whether or not e-therapy is "ethical" has been the subject of many heated debates in the mental health community. Over the years, the quality of this debate has changed substantially. In the early years, the debate was sharply divided between an outraged majority who proclaimed that the practice was completely unethical and dangerous and, an equally impassioned minority who were actually engaged in it and witnessing e-therapy's potential to help.

After years of observing the e-therapy field, I can say that psychotherapists who practice on the Internet are among the most ethical people I know. They are skilled professionals who take their sacred duty as healers very seriously. They don't harm people; they help people. They are pioneers who saw a need, took a risk, and reached out to help. They are forging this new field because they believe that it is helping people.

A few mental health professionals still feel very strongly, however, that it is not ethical for psychotherapists to attempt to treat people on the Internet. These critics speak from the heart. They say they represent the best interest of consumers. Many believe that e-therapy will not help, and some believe that it will harm. They present many "what if" scenarios that turn out badly. Considering my own highly successful experience with e-therapy, one might think I would speak out against these opponents of e-therapy, but one would be wrong. I truly respect their concern. Their cautionary voices are essential to the exploration of this new frontier.

It is most certainly true that not all therapists have an aptitude for counseling over the Internet, and just as indisputable that e-therapy is not appropriate for every patient. Some "what if" scenarios are examples of situations in which e-therapy is contraindicated. On the other hand, there are other situations in which e-therapy is absolutely the best alternative available.

Unfortunately, it is easy to get sidetracked. Is e-therapy really therapy? Is e-therapy better than regular therapy? Will e-therapy replace regular therapy? These are the wrong questions. Of course, e-therapy is never going to replace traditional therapy. And even if e-therapy is not "real" therapy, there is no question that it can be very helpful. People will continue seeking advice on the Internet. If ethical, credentialed, reputable e-therapists aren't available, some people will take the advice of whoever is. Some people will have no other choice. Given this reality, I think ethical therapists practically have a duty to be available on the Internet.

Today, having accumulated so much positive anecdotal evidence, discussion has largely shifted from "whether" to "how." Now most professionals wonder not "Should e-therapy be offered?" but "How should e-therapy be offered to be most effective and ethical?" Every day, hundreds, maybe thousands, of people form relationships with professional psychotherapists via the Internet. Some are profoundly helped by this process; some are not. Psychotherapists must continue to explore the dangers and opportunities in this new frontier.

It is also vitally important for consumers to participate in this process. Without input from knowledgeable consumers, mental health professionals cannot fully know how e-therapy is or isn't helping. We consumers must take responsibility for differentiating between what helps and what doesn't, and find the courage to voice what we think is right or wrong. If e-therapy helps people who otherwise would not be helped, we need to tell the critics that. We need to speak up, and professionals need to listen.

The creative tension must continue. Those involved in this new field must be reminded of the risks and of the benefits. All voices must be heard—those of critics and proponents, e-therapists and e-patients. We must not allow anyone to be silenced. If cyberspace does anything, it helps people to speak more freely.

All they need is someone to listen.

Reference

U.S. Department of Health and Human Services. (1999). *Mental health: A report of the Surgeon General*. Rockville, MD: Author. [Online]. Available: www.surgeongeneral.gov/library/mentalhealth/home.html

INDEX

ABCs of e-therapy, 203–4
Abnormal Involuntary Movement Scale (AIMS)
    evaluating video equipment's transmission to
        enable examination using, 72
    reliability of, in telemedicine application, 82
    reliability of videoconferencing for assessing,
        research in, 80
acceptance, of telemedicine, NARBHA, 84
access to care
    behavioral health services, problems of
        delivery in rural areas, 70
    universal, future of, 10
    through videoconferencing, 81
accuracy
    of information from the Internet, assessing,
        18–19
    in traditional and Internet publishing, 10–11
addiction, to the Internet, 142
addresses, standardization of, 2
adjunct services
    use of e-mail
        case examples of, xi–xiii
        negative consequences of, 64–65
        in therapy for anorexia nervosa, 41–47
    use by mental health professionals, 207
administration
    of scattered service sites through
        videoconferencing, 79
    services in the e-health industry, 167
Advanced Research Projects Agency (ARPA),
        origins of the Internet in, 2
advertising, of Web sites, 12
    direct-to-consumer pharmaceutical
        promotion, 181
advisor, therapist as, 148
Agras, W. S., 66
Ainsworth, M., 12, 96, 153
Algazy, J. I., 182

Almer, E., 183
American Counseling Association (ACA),
        standards for online counseling, 153,
        160
American Medical Association (AMA)
    guidelines for e-therapists, 178
    guidelines for ethical practice, 152
    Medem Web site of, 167
American Medical Informatics Association
        (AMIA), 178
    guidelines on e-mail in clinical and
        administrative work, 140
American Psychiatric Association (APA)
    guidance for e-therapists, 178
    guidelines for ethical practice, 152
    study of telepsychiatry, 167–68
    Web sites through, 65–66
American Psychological Association (APA)
    on the efficacy of psychotherapy, 93
    Ethics Committee, 152
    guidelines on online services, 153–54
American Telemedicine Association (ATA), 140
America Online (AOL), membership
        requirement for participation in private
        chat rooms, 100
AmericasDoctor site, xxiii–xxiv, 39
amnesia, case example, questions about, on the
        Internet, 33–34
Andrews, B., 33
anonymity, of patients in e-therapy
    legal issues arising from, 178
    power of, xxi–xxii
anorexia nervosa, e-mail support for outpatient
        treatment of, 39–68
Appel, R. D., 152
Arizona Department of Health Services,
        Division of Behavioral Health Services,
        72

217

"Ask the Expert" site of Mental Health
Infosource, 24–25
"Ask Uncle Ezra," place in the history of online
mental health advice, 205–9
Asmonga, D. D., 152
attachment, questions about, for an Internet
"expert," 34–35
Australian Psychological Society (APS),
standards for online counseling, 153
authority, the therapist as, in the information
age, 148
autonomy, in the virtual world, therapists'
understanding of, 139

Baars, B. J., 33
Baer, L., 81
Barak, A., 92–93
Bates, D. W., 179, 180
Bauer, K., 177
Baur, C., 11, 81
behavioral health services, delivery of, problems
in rural areas, 70
benefits
of adjunctive e-mail, 62–64
from the online provision of mental health
services, evaluating, 155
Bergh, C., 66
Bergman, A., 133
Berland, G. K., 182
Berners-Lee, T., 3
Bertsch, T., 71
bias, in Internet-based advice, 143
Bienz v. Central Suffolk Hospital, on
physician-patient relationship, 176
Black, M., 182
Bleger, J., xix
Bloom, J. W., 153
Blubaugh, D., ix
Board of Medical Examiners, Texas, on
prescription in Internet practice, 174
Bonsch, C., 66
Boole, G., 15
Boolean logic, for searching the Web, 15–18
Boulding, M. E., 159
Boyer, C., 152
Brennan, T. A., 178
Brewin, D. R., 33
Broder, M. S., 182
Brown, R. K., 160
buddy list, AOL, for creating private chat rooms,
100
bulimia nervosa, self-help guidance for, 66
Burdick, E., 179
Bureau of Health Services, Michigan, licensing
boards of, 170

Burgiss, S. G., 86
Burns, C., 81
business-to-consumer services, 167
Butler, D., 18

care. see access to care, quality of care
Carey, B., 187
case examples
of adjunctive e-mail, xi–xiii
from "Ask the Expert," x–xi, 28–35
of chat room therapy, xiv–xv, 100–133
of co-management of a patient with e-mail,
58–59
of community telepsychiatry, xiii–xiv
of e-mail
for adjunctive therapy in anorexia nervosa,
41–47
to communicate with family members,
55–58
for monitoring therapy from a distance,
42–51
of long-term chat room therapy, 128–33
of short-term chat room therapy, 110–28
Caspi v. Microsoft Network, 184
catalogs, structure and content of, 14
chat room therapy, 92–135
competence of therapist in, 93–94
confidentiality in, 95–96
"Cyberpsych" Internet Relay Chat service, 206
distraction in, 97–98
identity of clients in, 94–95
levels of care in, 98–99
licensure in, 96
and long-term therapy, example, 128–33
and nonverbal information, 94
oversight in, 96, 98–99
PayPal, 100
research in, 92–93
and short-term therapy, example, 110–28
suicide, managing threats of in, 96–97
timing of interactions in, disrupted turn
adjacency, 99–100
triage and referral in, example, 101–10
Childress, C., 92, 94–96
Chin, T., 181
Chong, N. S. T., 19
clients. see consumers, patients
clinical practice
and care, principles of, and telemedicine,
85–88
flexibility in, xvi, 137–38
and potential of the Internet, ix–xxiv
principles for, xv–xvi
principles for guiding the practice of
e-therapy, 136–49

respect in, 138–39
responsibility in, xvi, 141
and utilization of NARBHA Net, 74
clinicians. *see* physicians, professionals, therapists
collaboration
online, advantages of, 162
by the therapist, 148
co-management of a patient, with e-mail, 58–59
commerce, selling keywords in search reports, 18
Community Partnership of Southern Arizona,
network of teleconference clinic sites, 72
community program, in telepsychiatry, 69–91
competence
in clinical practice, xvi, 139–41
ethical duty of the therapist to limit advice to
areas of, 156
therapist's, in chat room therapy, 93–94
confidentiality
in chat room therapy, 95–96
protecting, ethical principle, 157
in telemedical practice, 86
in the virtual world, therapists' understanding
of, 139
see also, privacy
conflict of interest, in advertising on medical
advice sites, 169–70
Constantinou, P. S., 66
consultation, in videoconferencing networks, 76
Consumer Reports, survey on efficacy of
psychotherapy, 93
consumers
empowering, with information from the
Internet, 6
Federal Trade Commission, U.S., authority in
protecting consumer privacy, 170
free market, and patient protection, issues in
regulation, 160
information for, 4–5, 203–4
interactions with mental health professionals,
types of, 206–7
satisfaction of, with e-therapy, survey results,
208
see also, patients
continuing education credits, medical, network
connection for psychiatric grand rounds
to earn, 72
continuity of care, in rural areas, utilizing
telemedicine, 81
correctional institutions, services to inmates of,
80
cost
of e-therapy, information for the client about,
212–13
of telemedicine, 83–84
see also, payment

countertransference, in telemedicine, 87–88
crisis intervention, with e-mail, 59–61
Cukor, P., 81
Cullen, D. J., 179
cyberchondria, 142
CyberDocs site, 39
"Cyberpsych" Internet Relay Chat service, 206

danger, in Internet practice, 151–53
see also, problems
data, sources of, "reader beware" in using, 4
see also, accuracy
Deering, M. J., 11, 81
Delamothe, T., 182
demographics, of NARBHA Net clients, 75
Department of Justice (DOJ), U.S., on Internet
prescriptions, 174
Deutsch, H., 160
Dev, P., 66
Digital Library Initiative, U.S., on the
organization of information on the
Internet, 13–14
Dimmick, S. L., 86
direct-to-consumer pharmaceutical promotion,
181
disinhibition, online, 195–96
distance learning, 19–20
distraction, in chat room therapy, from the lack
of an obvious client, 97–98
Ditton, T., 94, 133
Doctor Global, as an example of good e-therapy
practice, xvi, 143–45
Dodd, P. W., 40
Douglas, R. M., 180
drugs
paroxetine, in anorexia nervosa, 42
specific, requesting information about from an
Internet "expert," 31–32
see also, medications
Dubler, N. N., 169
Dunham, P. J., 40

e-clinics, advent of, 207–8
education
academic programs online, 6
versus medical practice, in answering online
questions, 25
of patients, by online "experts," 28, 37–38
training using videoconferences, 78–79
see also, "experts," information
e-health, 166–68
and quality of care, 181
Eldredge, K. L., 66
Elias, M., 168
Elliott, M. N., 182

Ellsworth, C., 40
e-mail
    for anorexia nervosa outpatient treatment
        support, 39–68
    and the co-management of a patient, 58–59
    and crisis intervention, 59–61
    emotional value of, to patients, 62–64
    establishing a therapist-patient relationship
        through, 176–77
    evaluating responses from patients, 64
    evolution in use of, in treating anorexia
        nervosa, 40–41
    fees for outpatient care via, 66
    and the function of the Internet, 2
    groups for people with eating disorders, 66–67
    guidelines for utilizing in therapy, 160–61
    for monitoring food intake, 51–54
    monitoring therapy from a distance via, 42–51
    privacy of, for therapy, 202
    problems in e-mail practice, scenario for
        circumventing, 162–63
    professional issues in therapy, 65–66
    therapy, adjunctive use in, 41–47
    use of in transition between care providers,
        54–55
Emanuel, E. J., 169
emergencies, responding to
    e-therapists responsibility for, 184
    for patients at a geographic distance, xvii, 157
e-patient, life as an, 194–215
e-publication, advantages and limitations of,
    10–12
    see also, publishing
equipment, video
    reliability of, for telemedicine systems, 86–87
    for telemedicine systems, 72–73
Eriksson, M., 66
error, medical. see medical error
    Estates of Morgan v. Fairfield Family Counseling
        Center, 183
e-therapy
    ABCs of, 203–4
    criteria for choosing, 210
    future of, 145–48
    holding environment in, xii
    implications of legal issues for, xvii–xix,
        166–99
    legal issues in the growth of, 170–87
    limitations of, informing patients about,
        212–13
    opportunity for, 151–53
    practice, example of, 143–45
    presence of therapist in, xii
    problems with, 142–43
        a scenario, 150–51

promise of, versus legal and ethical questions,
    187–88
scheduling and payment, structure of, 156
surveying the field of, 204–9
tradeoffs in, 159–60
triage and referral, example, 101–10
turnaround time and, 55
ethics
    for e-therapy, 213–15
    professional, for e-therapy, i–xvii, 150–65
    traditional guidelines for provision of mental
        health services, 152
evaluation
    of NARBHA Net, 81–84
    of the patient online, ethical standards, 156
evidence-based medicine
    Cochrane Library of, 6
    for decreasing medical error, 179–80
"experts," Internet
    the promise and perils of, 24–38
    disclaimer, for a Web site featuring an
        "expert," 27
    medications, requesting information about
        from, 31–32
    on St. John's Wort (hypericum), 31–32
expert systems, for monitoring quality of care,
    179–80
extensible markup language (XML), 20–21
extension, of Web-based information, 10
Eysenbach, G., 177

family, communication with hospitalized
        members by e-mail, 55–58
Federal Trade Commission (FTC), U. S.
    authority in protecting consumer privacy,
        170
    on fraudulent health products marketed on
        the Internet, 182
fees, for outpatient e-mail care, 66
    see also, payments
Feist, J., 205
Fenichel, M., 93, 153
Ferguson, T., 137
file transfer protocol (FTP), and the function of
        the Internet, 2
"Find-A-Therapist," 208
Fine, S. F., 12
Fink, J., 94
Food and Drug Administration (FDA), U.S.
    on fraudulent health products marketed on
        the Internet, 182
    Internet pharmacy regulation by, 173
food intake, monitoring by e-mail, 51–54
    Frakes v. Cardiology Consultants, 179
Franklin, D., 153

free market, and patient protection, issues in
    regulation, 160
Freudenheim, M., 179
Fugh-Berman, A., 32
future
    of e-therapy, 145–48
    of online information, 19–21
    of videoconferencing in rural areas, 79–80

Gagliardi, A., 182
Gawande, A. A., 180
Gibson, S., xiii
Goldberg, I., 205
Gooden v. Tips, 175
grand rounds
    psychiatric, continuing education credits for
        network attendance at, 72
    webcasts of, 6
Gray, J. A. M., 179–80
Greater Arizona Training Alliance, 79
Greene, J., 166
Greist, J., 153
Grohol, J., 93, 96, 153, 205
Gross, S. J., 92, 94–95, 96
guidance
    for e-patients, 209–11
    for e-therapists, 211–13
guidelines
    American Counseling Association (ACA), for
        online counseling, 153, 160
    American Medical Association (AMA), for
        e-therapists, 178
    American Medical Association (AMA), for
        ethical practice, 152
    American Medical Informatics Association
        (AMIA), on e-mail in clinical and
        administrative work, 140
    American Psychiatric Association (APA), for
        e-therapists, 178
    American Psychiatric Association (APA), for
        ethical practice, 152
    Australian Psychological Society (APS), for
        online counseling, 153
    clinical principles for practice of e-therapy,
        136–49
    clinical care, principles of, and telemedicine,
        85–88
    ethical standards for the evaluation of the
        patient online, 156
    Health on the Net, 145, 152, 154
    Hi-Ethics, Inc., for provision of health
        information online, 152
    limitations of suggested principles for
        e-therapy, 158–59
    for terminology used by e-therapists, 157–58

for therapists, 211–13
    traditional, for provision of mental health
        services, 152
Gusella, J., 40

Hall, P., 19
Halmi, K. A., 66
Hamilton, S., 133
Hartley, P., 66
Hartwell-Walker, M., 92
Haynes, R. B., 179–80
Health and Human Services (HHS), U. S.
    Department of, reducing administrative
    costs of insurance with digital health
    records, 184–85
HealthConnect, consumer control over
    electronic health records through,
    145–46
Healtheon Corporation, survey on e-mail
    communication between physicians and
    patients, 39
Health Insurance Portability and Accountability
    Act (HAPPY), xix, 178, 184–85
    on patient confidentiality, 65–66
Health on the Net (HON) Code of Conduct for
    Medical and Health Web Sites, 145
Health on the Net Foundation (HON)
    guidelines for provision of health information
        online, 152, 154
    safety and reliability of Web-based medical
        information, 182
health records. see records
Hebert, L., 178
HelpHorizons.com, 208
heuristic responses, to people seeking Internet
    medical advice, 26
Hiatt, H. H., 178
Hickey, M., 179
Hi-Ethics, Inc.
    guidelines for provision of health information
        online, 152
    on safety and reliability of Web-based medical
        information, 182
Hilts, P. J., 182
holding environment, in e-therapy, xii
Holmes, L. G., 66, 92, 94, 96
    "Shareware Psychological Consultation" of,
        205
home health care, provision of psychiatric
    services through videoconferencing,
    79–80
hopelessness, 195
Hordern, B. B., 183
Horton, F., 12, 13
Hsiung, R. C., 153, 154

Hubbard, S., 12
Hughes, R. S., 152
Hurshman, A., 40
Hussain, H., 182
Hyler, S. E., 1
hypericum (St. John's Wort), information about, from an Internet "expert," 31–32
hypertext, and user friendly Web use, 3
hypertext markup language (HTML), 9
　upgrading, 20–21

identity, of clients in chat room therapy, 94–95
　see also, anonymity
Infodynamics, Second Law of, x
information
　assessing, on the Internet, 18–19
　accumulation of, 9
　availability of, 7–12
　client-provided, analysis of, 138
　continuous access to, and sense of timelessness on the Web, 19–21
　Digital Library Initiative, U.S., 13–14
　distance learning, 19–20
　evolution of transfer of, 7–10
　explosion of, in mental health, 1–23
　extension of via of via Web, 10
　finding, 12–13
　future of online, 19–21
　as a goal in Internet use, 3
　impact of innovation on, 19–20
　integrity of, as presented on the Web, 18–19
　literacy in handling, 12–13
　about mental illness, online, 4
　and metadata, 21
　nonverbal, and chat room demeanor, 94
　online, x
　　types of, 4–7
　overload, 21
　about patient, screening and verifying online, 152–53
　quality of, in e-health, 181–82
　quantity of, 12
　seeking on Internet, regarding illness, 5
　therapist-provided, quality of, 212
　validation of, from the Internet, 18–19
　videoconferencing among staff and client, 75
　see also, media, publishing
informed consent
　form
　　for telemedicine participation, 90–91
　　for videoconference use, 74
　principle of, in the online provision of mental health services, xvii, 154–55, 177–78
informediaries, 167
insurance. see malpractice insurance

interactive media, on the Web, 3
International Society for Mental Health Online (ISMHO), 153, 208, 213
　guidance for e-therapists, 178
　and the Psychiatric Society of Informatics (PSI), xvi, 93
Internet
　addiction to, 142
　danger of, 151–53
　and real-world practice, 137–41
　self-care, promoting by means of, 146–47
　and the World Wide Web, 1–2
Internet Healthcare Coalition (IHC)
　guidelines for provision of health information online, 152
　on safety and reliability of Web-based medical information, 182
Internet therapy, ABCs of, 203–9
interpersonal issues, in e-therapy, legal, 175–78

Jadad, A. R., 182
Jane Doe One v. Oliver, 182
Johnson, T., 37
Joy v. Eastern Maine Medical Center, 175

Kane, B., 154, 178, 185
Kanouse, D. E., 182
Kashishian v. Port, 180
Kelman, C. W., 180
Kennedy, R., x, 1
Kesselman, M., 153
Kiesler, S., 40
King, S. A., 3, 64, 160, 162
Kirk, P., 153
Kleefield, S., 179
Klyce, B., x
Kottler, J. A., 133
Kramer, T., 1
Kravitz, R. L., 182
Kraybill, J., 153
Krebs, B., 182
Kuszler, P. C., 176

Labott, S. M., 33
Laird, N. M., 178, 179
Landro, L., 166, 167, 181
Lara, M., 182
Lasswitz, K., 19
Lawthers, A. G., 178
Leahy, L., 81
Leape, L. L., 178, 179
Leavitt, R., 33
legal issues
　regarding anonymity of patients, 178
　in the growth of e-therapy, 170–87

implications, of e-therapy, xvii–xix, 166–93
  questions about the Internet "expert," 24–28
  refining online suggestions to meet, 26–27
  requirements for therapists, 156
  see also, liability systems, licensure
Lester, D., 40
levels of care, for chat room therapy, 98–99
liability systems, in e-health practices, 169
licensure
  in chat room therapy, 96
  in e-therapy, 171
  issues in, xxi
  indeterminate location of e-therapy and, 172–73
  multiple licensing boards and the Bureau of
    Health Services of Michigan, 170
Lim, R., 153
limitations
  of e-therapy, informing patients about,
    212–13
  of suggested principles for e-therapy therapy,
    158–59
Lindberg, G., 66
literacy, in information handling, 12–13
Little Colorado Behavioral Health Centers, 69,
    74–78
Litwin, E., 40
Localio, A. R., 178
location
  of e-therapy, 158
  indeterminate, of e-therapy, and licensure,
    172–73
Lombard, M., 94, 133
long-term therapy, chat room example, 128–33

McGlynn, E. A., 182
McGovern, K., 33
McGuire, T., 40
MacMillan, R., 173, 175
Maheu, M., 96
Mahler, M., xii
Mahrer, A. R., 133
malpractice insurance
  role of practice guidelines in defining, 179–81
  for telemedicine consultation, 172
Mankita, S., 93, 99
marketing, deceptive, on the Internet, 143
Marshall, S., 183
Matsushita Electric Corporation of America, 167
Maurer, G., 66
MedCertain, rating of the quality of Web-based
    medical information, 182
Medem, 167
media
  published, comparisons of, 8–9
  the World Wide Web place in, 2–4
  see also, information, publishing

medical error, concerns over, xviii, 178–79
medications
  automation of prescription, 178–79
  Department of Justice, U.S., on Internet
    prescriptions, 174direct-to-consumer
    pharmaceutical promotion, 181
  dispensing, based on Internet consultation,
    174–75
  Food and Drug Administration, U.S., Internet
    pharmacy regulation by, 173
  online questions about, 28–30
  prescribing for telepsychiatry patients, 76
  prescribing on the Internet, 25–26, 172,
    173–74
  Texas Board of Medical Examiners, on
    prescription of in Internet practice,
    174
Medline, database of published material in
    medicine and health, 6
Medscape, medical and mental health
    information from, 7
megasites, medical, 7
Mental Health Clinic, of Global Doctor, 144
Mental Health Cyber-Clinic, 197–202
Mental Health Infosource, "Ask the Expert" site
    of, 24–25
mental illnesses, online information about, 4
metadata, tagging information to provide, 21
Metanoia.org, xx, 203–9
  listing of therapists, 93
Michigan, Bureau of Health Services of, multiple
    licensing boards, 170
Microsoft, on e-health systems, 167
Miller v. Sullivan, xviii
  on patient-physician relationship, 176
Mitchell, D. L., 40, 159–60
Mitchell, J. E., 66
Morabito, C., 81
Morales, L. S., 182
Moreggi, D., 160, 162
Morley, S., xiii, 72
Mount, C. D., 180
multiple treatment providers, 156
Muñoz, J. A., 182
Murphy, L. J., 40, 159–60

Nadler, 133
NARBHA Net, xiii–xiv
  and acceptance of telemedicine, 84
  description of equipment selection and
    utilization, 72–74
  financing of, by tobacco tax revenues, 72
  technical description of, 88–90
  see also, Northern Arizona Regional Behavioral
    Health Authority

National Alliance for the Mentally Ill (NAMI),
   30
National Association of Boards of Pharmacy
   (NABP), 175
National Board for Certified Counselors
   (NBCC), 140
   standards for e-therapy, 153–54
National Depressive and Manic Depressive
   Association (NDMDA), 36
National Electronic Health Records Taskforce,
   Australia, 145
National Library of Medicine (NLM), catalogs
   online, 6
Navajo Indian Reservation, of Apache County
   Colorado, 74
Needham, E., 206
Negroponte, N., 62–63, 65
netcasts. see webcasts
Newhouse, J. P., 178
New York University, Web site offering
   screening tests for psychiatric disorders,
   30–31
Northern Arizona Regional Behavioral Health
   Authority (NARBHA), 69
   history of, 70
   see also, NARBHA Net

object constancy, of the therapist, in e-therapy,
   xii
Office for the Advancement of Telehealth
   (OAT), 168
Ohio Department of Rehabilitation, study of
   suicidal clients, 97
on-call coverage, with videoconferencing,
   80
Operation Cure All, 182
operators, Boolean, for searching, 15–16
Orey, H., webmaster, "Ask the Expert," 25
outpatient treatment, of anorexia nervosa, e-mail
   to support, 39–68
oversight, in chat room therapy, 96
   by the client, 98–99

Park-Cunningham, R., 153
patients
   e-mail communication with physicians, 39
   empowering with access to digital health
     records, 20
   guidance for, 209–11
   identity of, xxii–xxiii
   online, screening and verifying information
     about, 152–53
   perspective of, xix–xx
   records of, online, availability to the
     physician, 10

relationship with therapist, xviii, 175–77
   see also, consumers
payment
   fees for outpatient e-mail care, 66
   for online services, client's questions about,
     211
   PayPal, for receiving payment for chat room
     therapy, 100
   scheduling and payment, structure of, 156
   see also, cost, reimbursement
Pederson, C., 67
Perez v. Wyeth Laboratories, 181
Perls, F., 34
personalization, of Web interfaces, 21
Petersen, L. A., 179
Pew Internet & American Life Project, on
   Internet users' accessing health
   information, 4–5
physicians,
   use of Internet and e-mail, 39
   see also, professionals, therapists
Pies, R., xi, xxiii, 25
Pinal Gila Behavioral Health Association
   (PGBHA), linkage with Behavioral
   Health Services in Phoenix, Arizona, 72
Pine, F., 133
Pool, R., 13
Posner, E. M., 173
Poulos, S. T., 64
prescriptions. see medications
presence
   of the therapist, in e-therapy, xii
   in video- or computer- mediated experience,
     94
principles, for providing online mental health
   services, 153–57
   see also, guidelines
privacy
   of electronic information, xviii, 185–87
   and e-mail, respect for clients in utilizing, 139
   of e-mail for therapy, example, 202
   in e-therapy, acknowledging, 155, 211
   user concerns about, Pew Internet & American
     Life Project data, 4–5
privileging requirements, institutional, and
   online consulting, 172
professional associations, Web sites of, 6–7
professionals
   communication among, about a patient, 48
   information for, from the Internet, 6
   interactions with mental health consumers,
     types of, 206–7
   see also, physicians, therapists
profile, on America Online (AOL), therapist's
   creation of, 100–133

protocols, standardization of, 2
  see also, guidelines
psyche, global technological, 3
Psychiatric Society for Informatics (PSI),
    153
publishing
  accuracy of, in traditional form and on the
      Internet, 10–11
  cycles, traditional and Internet, 11
  e-publication, advantages and limitations of,
      10–12
  standards, for Internet, 11
  see also, information, media
Puyol, J. A., 182

quality of care
  and e-health, 181–84
  legal issues for e-therapists in telemedicine,
      Arizona experience, 183–84
  and risk avoidance, proactive, 180
  and technology, in traditional practice, xviii,
      178–84
  in telemedicine, Arizona experience, 81–83
questions, for the therapist, Internet, 24–28

Rathner, G., 66
real-world practice, the Internet in, 137–41
Reason, J., 179
recommendations
  prescriptive, 26
  proscriptive, 26
records
  digital, 20
  maintenance of, by the therapist, 157
  medical, managing for NARBHA clients
      referred for inpatient care, 75–76
  online, availability to the physician, 10
  privacy of note from therapy sessions, 187
  reducing administrative costs of insurance
      with digital records, 184–85
regulation
  of health care providers, challenges with
      e-commerce, 169
  legal issues and growth of e-therapy, xviii,
      170–75
reimbursement, for telemedicine services,
    172
  see also, cost, payment
relationships
  dishonest, on the Web, 143
  therapist-client, searching for, 196–98
  therapist-patient, xviii, 175–77
research
  on the accuracy of online health information,
      182

in chat room therapy, 92–93
  on the efficacy of psychotherapy, 93
  in e-therapy, building a database for, 141
  on outpatient treatment for anorexia nervosa,
      66
  in telemedicine, University of Arizona
      Telemedicine Program, 80
residential treatment facilities, communication
    with the home community using
    videoconferencing, 77
respect, in clinical practice, 138–39
  on the Internet, xvi
responsibility, in clinical practice, xvi, 141
Richardson, W. S., 179–80
risk
  avoidance of, proactive, and quality of care,
      180
  from the online provision of mental health
      services, evaluating, 155
  safeguards from, in the online provision of
      mental health services, 155–56
Robson, D., 152
Robson, M., 152
Rodriguez, J. C., 160
Rogers, E. M., xxi
Romeo-Wolff, C., xiii
Rosenberg, W. M. C., 179–80
Rosenthal, R. M., 153
Rosik, C. H., 160
Rothchild, E., 65
Russell, B., 2
Rust, J. N., 153

Sackett, D. L., 179–80
safeguards. see risk
"safe text," in e-mail therapy, 65–66
Samaritans, 36, 206
Sanderson, W. C., 93
Sands, D. Z., 154, 177, 178, 185
scheduling, flexibility in, in the virtual world,
    138
Scherer, J. R., 152
Schulman, C. E., 65, 153
Schwarz, M. F., 18
Scribbins, K., 186
search engines
  categories of, 14
  magic of, 13–14
  metasearch, 14
searching
  limiting by means of target attributes, 17–18
  use of parentheses for refining, 17
  techniques for, 15–18
  terms for, 15
  for a therapist-client relationship, 196–98

seclusion of patients, complying with medical
    supervision regulations with
    videoconferencing, 80
security, standards proposed by U. S.
    Department of Health and Human
    Services, xviii, 185
Seger, D. L., 179
Selby, M., 152
self-analysis, requests for tools for, on the
    Internet, 30–31
self-care, promoting by means of Internet
    resources, 146–47
    see also, quality of care
self-determination, in the virtual world,
    therapists' understanding of, 139
Seligman, M. E. P., 93
Shapiro, D. E., 65, 153
shareware psychological consultation, 205–6
Sharpe, T., 66
Shea, B., 179
Sherman, C., 66
short-term therapy, chat room example, 110–28
    see also, e-therapy
Shulman, R., 96
Siegel, J., 40
Silverman, R. D., 171
Smith, G. T., 86
Smith, L. R., 180
Smith, R., 146
Sodersten, P., 66
Sollner, W., 66
Sommers, D., 206
Spielberg, A. R., 65, 177, 178, 185
stalking, on the Web, 143
standard operating procedure, in e-therapy, xvii,
    156–57
Stern, D. M., xv
Stofle, G., xiv–xv, 92, 93, 133, 153
Stroh, M., 39
structure
    of health care delivery, changes with
        e-therapy, 168–69
    for Web pages, 9
suicide
    Internet "expert" answers to questions about,
        35–37
    managing threats of, in chat room therapy,
        96–97
    Ohio Department of Rehabilitation, study of
        suicidal clients, 97
Suler, J., 92, 93
Sullivan, L., 138
Supervision
    of e-therapists, 133
    Doctor Global example, 144–45

support groups
    international, online, 195
    "Walkers in Darkness," example of, 205

tables of content, online, 12
tagging, of information with basic descriptive
    material, 21
Tapellini, D., 179
Tarasoff v. Regents of the University of California, xxii,
    183
Taylor, C. B., 66
technology, and quality of care in traditional
    practice, 178–84
Teich, J. M., 179
telemedicine
    acceptance of, and NARBHA, 84
    boundaries of, 87–88
    confidentiality in, 86
    and continuity of care, in rural areas, 81
    and countertransference, 87–88
    defined, Arizona statutes, 171
    equipment for telemedicine systems, 72–73,
        86–87
    factors driving establishment of, 70–72
    and informed consent for participation, 90–91
    transference in, 87–88
    transmission quality, and satisfaction with,
        85
    see also, telepsychiatry, videoconferencing
telepsychiatry
    American Psychiatric Association study of,
        167–68
    defined for discussion of legal issues, 166
    NARBHA as model community program in,
        69–91
    see also, telemedicine, videoconferencing
telnet, function of the Internet, 2
terminology, of guidelines for e-therapists,
    157–58
Terry, N. P., xvii–xix, 169–70, 180, 182, 187
tests, screening for psychiatric disorders, offered
    by New York University Web site, 30–31
therapists
    as advisors, 148
    authority of, in the information age, 148
    autonomy of, understanding of by, in the
        virtual world, 139
    competence in chat room therapy, 93–94
    computer skills of, 140–41
    evaluating
        before entering a relationship, 210
        in e-therapy, 155
        guidance for, 211–13
        intuition of, 200–201
        object constancy of, in e-therapy, xii

presence of, in e-therapy, xii questions for,
    regarding Internet, 24–28
relationship with patient, xviii, 175–77
responses to e-mail from patients, 64
responsibility for responding to emergencies,
    184
roles of, defining in the information age, 148
strength of, 200–201
supervision of, 133
training of, 133
see also, physicians, professionals
Tice, N., 153
timelessness, continuous access to information
    on the Web, 19–21
Torello, G., 153
Tracy v. Merrell Dow Pharmaceuticals, 180
training, of e-therapists, 133
transference, in telemedicine, 87–88
transmission quality, video system, and
    satisfaction with telemedicine, 85
treatment team, presence at client
    videoconferencesamong psychiatrists
    and patients, 83
triage and referral, in single-session chat room
    therapy, example, 101–10
trust, in e-therapist and client relationship, 203,
    212–13
Tunkl v. Regents of the University of California, 184
Turkel, S., 40, 63
turnaround time, in e-therapy, 155

uniform resource locators (URLs), 3
university Web sites, uses of for library and
    research information, 6
utilization rates, for NARBHA, 73–74

values, of professional ethics, 151–52
Vander Vliet, M., 179
Vardell, M., 153
Verified Internet Pharmacy Practice Sites
    (VIPPS), 175
videoconferencing
    and access to care, 81
    and administration of scattered service sites,
        79
    among Arizona State Hospital and regional
        agencies, 77
    and consultation, 76
    educational training via, 78–79
    future of, in rural areas, 79–80
    and home health care, provision of psychiatric
        services, 79–80
    and informed consent, 74
    management of a videoconference network,
        80

on-call coverage and, 80
to provide access to psychiatry in medically
    underserved areas, 69
between residential treatment facilities and
    home communities, 77
and the seclusion of patients, complying with
    medical supervision regulations, 80
among staff and client, 75
treatment team, presence of during, 83
visiting with family by means of, 78
see also, telemedicine, telepsychiatry
visiting, with family through videoconferencing,
    78

Walker-Schmucker, W., 153
"Walkers in Darkness" support group, 205
walking wounded, communication among on the
    Web, 196
Walter, M. H., 66
Warner, T., 67
Warren, B., 1
Watkins, K. E., 182
Web. see Internet
webcasts, of grand rounds, 6
webmaster, for an Internet medical advice site,
    25
WebMD, 39, 167
Web sites
    of publishers, 6–7
    readership of, building, 11
    of therapists, 65–66
weight, monitoring diet in, with e-mail,
    51–53
Weiler, P. C., 178
Weinstock, L., 81
Wells, H. G., 22
Wells, J., 185
Welsh, T. S., 86
Williams v. America Online, 184
Wilson, G., 40
Winnicott, D. W., xii
Winzelberg, A. J., 66
wireless markup language (WML), 10
Woody, S., 93
World Wide Web. see Internet
Worona, S., 205
Wurman, R. S., 12, 21
Wylie, M., 93

Yager, J., xii–xiii, 67
Yank, H., 182
Yellowlees, P. M., xv–xvi, 139, 140,
    142–43

Zarate, C. A., 81